AF781012

CANCER IN CHILDHOOD

JOHN O. GODDEN, M.D.
EDITOR

Springer Science+Business Media, LLC

Proceedings of the 17th Clinical Conference of the Ontario Cancer Treatment and Research Foundation

© Springer Science+Business Media New York 1973
Originally published by Ontario Cancer Treatment and Research Foundation in 1973
Softcover reprint of the hardcover 1st edition 1973

ISBN 978-1-4684-2072-2 ISBN 978-1-4684-2070-8 (eBook)
DOI 10.1007/978-1-4684-2070-8

Library of Congress Catalog Card Number 73-15003
All Rights Reserved

It is illegal to reproduce any portion of this book without special arrangement with the publishers. Reproduction of this material without authorization by any duplication process whatsoever is a violation of copyright.

FOREWORD

Viewed as contributions to continuing medical education, many scientific meetings disappoint because, although program committees plan with care, bring together excellent faculty and expose them to their peers, to other physicians and to house staff, the effect is evanescent. Meetings expend much professional time and public funds to stimulate the relatively few who attend. Hence the dictum "Hold a symposium and reach a few hundred; circulate a proceedings and reach the world."

Despite this dictum, many organizers of scientific meetings shy away from the publication of proceedings, insisting that teachers will not participate if they have to prepare publishable manuscripts and, if they do agree to prepare them, will delay for months or, in some cases, will not come through at all. However, this is often a matter of organization and determination: e.g., some program chairmen make the payment of expenses and honoraria contingent upon receipt of a publishable manuscript. Cox and his colleagues in Australia went one better: they organized the First International Cancer Conference in Sydney in November 1972 and published a two-volume proceedings ("Melanoma and Skin Cancer" and "The Nature of Leukemia") *before* the meetings began. As Dr. Cox notes, "This preprinting of the full papers freed each speaker from the necessity of recounting large quantities of data so that each paper could be opened more rapidly and provocatively and then defended in discussion" (Report of the International Cancer Conference, *Med J Aust,* 1: 12-33, June 24, 1972). On his return from that meeting, R. M. Taylor, Secretary-General of the Union Internationale Contre le Cancer, one of the sponsors of the conference, spoke warmly of this meeting as "lively, provocative, and marked by enthusiastic audience participation".

During the last decade, major advances have been made in the management of cancer in childhood by surgery, irradiation and chemotherapy. The Ontario Cancer Treatment and Research Foundation devoted its 17th Clinical Conference to a general review of these advances and directed that this review be published and shared with a wide audience. Through their presentations, guest faculty from elsewhere in North America, Great Britain and France allow the readers of these proceedings to compare work done elsewhere with that being done at the Hospital for Sick Children, the Princess Margaret Hospital, and in the Foundation's Regional Cancer Treatment Centres.

These proceedings were made ready for the printer with the co-operation of the participants, by the tireless and skilled support of Dr. R. D. T. Jenkin, who rounded up the late manuscripts and prepared the discussions for final editing, and through the efficiency and thoroughness of Miss A. Thoral Maltby.

The Ontario Cancer Treatment and Research Foundation has sponsored clinical conferences annually from 1954 to 1968 and, then, subsequently in even years. Clinical cancer research conferences are now held in the "odd" years. In 1959, a Proceedings of the Sixth Clinical Conference "Cancer of the Cervix Uteri" was printed for "in house" distribution, and this policy was continued in the years following when volumes were distributed to cancer treatment centres and universities. In line with this tradition, the Foundation now offers the Proceedings of this 17th Clinical Conference as a contribution to continuing medical education in cancer in Ontario, elsewhere in Canada and outside our borders.

J. O. Godden, M.D., C.M., M.Sc.(Med.),
F.R.C.P.(C), M.A.(Educ. Th.),

Editor of Publications,
The Ontario Cancer Treatment
and Research Foundation

Contributing Institutions:

The Ontario Cancer Treatment and Research Foundation
The Princess Margaret Hospital
The Hospital for Sick Children

Program Committee

R. D. T. Jenkin (Chairman)
W. L. Donohue
P. D. McClure
M. J. Sonley
C. A. Stephens

Sessions held at

The Princess Margaret Hospital
500 Sherbourne Street
Toronto, Ontario

November 9-10, 1972

PARTICIPANTS

Guest Faculty

D. P. BURKITT, Medical Research Council, London, England.

G. J. D'ANGIO, Memorial Hospital for Cancer and Allied Diseases, New York.

J. M. M. DARTE, Charles A. Janeway Child Health Centre, St. John's, Newfoundland.

P. B. DENT, Department of Pediatrics, McMaster University, Hamilton.

C. E. KOOP, The Surgical Clinic for Children, Children's Hospital of Philadelphia.

D. E. MAGNER, Department of Pathology, University of Ottawa.

P. H. MORRIS JONES, Department of Child Health, St. Mary's Hospital, Manchester, England.

O. SCHWEISGUTH, Service de Pediatrie, Institut Gustave-Roussy, Villejuif, France.

L. F. SINKS, Department of Pediatrics, Roswell Park Memorial Institute, Buffalo, N.Y., U.S.A.

J. R. WILBUR, Children's Cancer Unit, Children's Hospital at Stanford, Palo Alto, Calif., U.S.A.

The Ontario Cancer Treatment and Research Foundation

D. E. CANNELL

E. N. MacKAY

A. H. SELLERS

The Princess Margaret Hospital

C. L. ASH

P. J. FITZPATRICK

R. D. T. JENKIN

M. J. SONLEY

The Hospital for Sick Children

S. H. EIN

P. C. FLEMING

M. H. FREEDMAN

D. C. HARWOOD-NASH

E. B. HENDRICK

H. J. HOFFMAN

R. D. JEFFS

J. KIKUCHI

J. F. K. MANCER

P. D. McCLURE

P. J. MIDDLETON

M. G. NORMAN

E. H. PAKES

E. F. SAUNDERS

C. A. STEPHENS

CONTENTS

Page

Welcome to the Conference
John R. Evans 1

Introduction to the Conference
J. M. M. Darte 3

Some Statistics on Childhood Cancer in Ontario
A. H. Sellers, E. N. MacKay and E. E. McLerie 5

The Manchester Children's Tumor Registry
P. H. Morris Jones 21

Wilms' Tumor: A Review of the Toronto Experience
M. J. Sonley 29

Neonatal Renal Tumors
J. F. K. Mancer 42

The National Wilms' Tumor Study: A Progress Report
Giulio J. D'Angio, et al 49

Panel on Wilms' Tumor
Moderator: J. M. M. Darte 55

Pathology of Tumors of the Testis in Children
Desmond Magner 60

Management of Embryonal Adenocarcinoma of the Testis in Childhood: an Analysis of 164 Cases
Robert D. Jeffs 68

Malignant Ovarian Tumors in Children
Sigmund H. Ein 78

Tumors of the Brain in Infancy and Childhood
E. Bruce Hendrick 83

Posterior Third Ventricle Tumors: Clinical Presentation and Role of Surgery
H. J. Hoffman and E. B. Hendrick 85

Neuroradiology of Posterior Third Ventricle Tumors
Derek Harwood-Nash 92

Pathology of Posterior Third Ventricle Masses
M. G. Norman 98

CONTENTS (continued)

Page

Radiotherapy of Posterior Third Ventricle Tumors
R. D. T. Jenkin 102

Panel on Management of Brain Tumors
Moderator: E. B. Hendrick 108

Histiocytosis X: Pathology
J. F. K. Mancer 113

Histiocytosis X: Management
M. J. Sonley and F. Ghavimi 128

Radiotherapy of Nasopharyngeal Angiofibroma
P. J. Fitzpatrick and W. D. Rider 139

Rhabdomyosarcoma in Childhood
R. D. T. Jenkin 157

Malignant Liver Tumors in Childhood
Sigmund H. Ein and Clinton A. Stephens 166

Neuroblastoma
Odile Schweisguth 171

Immunological Aspects of Neuroblastoma
Peter B. Dent 179

Operative Treatment of Neuroblastoma and Rhabdomyosarcoma
C. Everett Koop 185

Panel on Rhabdomyosarcoma and Neuroblastoma
Moderator: C. A. Stephens 191

Panel on Psychiatric Problems in the Management of Children with Malignancy
Moderator: M. J. Sonley 199

The Value of Laparotomy in the Staging of Hodgkin's Disease in Children
C. A. Stephens 202

Non-Hodgkin's Lymphoma in Children
Jordan R. Wilbur, Martin Mott, Margaret Sullivan and W. W. Sutow 204

Burkitt's Lymphoma
D. P. Burkitt 209

CONTENTS (continued)

Page

Panel on Malignant Lymphoma
Moderator: P. D. McClure 214

Controlled Clinical Trials in Leukemia in Children
L. F. Sinks 216

Viral Infections in Acute Leukemia
Peter J. Middleton 225

Bacterial Infection in Leukemia
P. C. Fleming 229

Methotrexate Toxicity
M. H. Freedman 223

Uric Acid Metabolism in Malignancy
E. Fred Saunders 236

Panel on Selected Problems in Management of Acute Leukemia
Moderator: P. D. McClure 240

Index 245

WELCOME TO THE CONFERENCE

JOHN R. EVANS, M.D., D.Phil. (Oxon.), F.A.C.P., F.R.C.P.(C)*

When it was suggested that I give words of wisdom someone who knows me well said "you can give the words – all the wisdom is in the audience". I appreciate Dr. Cannell's invitation to come and say a few words at the beginning of this conference. It is not just words of welcome but an expression of my own satisfaction at seeing emerge a concept which is extremely important; that is, the co-operation of people in many different disciplines in the control of malignant diseases and, particularly, the malignant diseases in childhood.

One might ask why a conference, which takes many people from different parts of the country and from many different disciplines, should be held to deal with what are often considered to be uncommon diseases. Perhaps even more important, one might ask if we are justified in assembling the expensive resources needed to deal with the cancers of childhood when they represent such a small fraction of total disease and disability in the community. But, you already know the answer to these questions. You are committed to the control of these diseases because, although they are uncommon, they cause tremendous suffering and are a leading cause of death in this age group. Furthermore, the management of these problems is complex, and few individuals possess all the resources necessary for the best care of the individual patient.

For some years now, I have been concerned about the separation of the several disciplines that are essential for the management of malignant disease. Thus it gives me particular pleasure to see this conference bring together people from the various disciplines involved in the management of malignant disease and the support of the patient and family. It is particularly satisfying to see that people from all parts of the country have come here to share their knowledge and experience. One would hope that this will result not only in pooling of information but also in a willingness to co-operate in the effective use of scarce and expensive resources for people in every part of Canada.

On behalf of the University of Toronto I would like to extend a warm welcome to you all. The Princess Margaret Hospital, with its unusual resources, also welcomes you. You will contribute to its programs by the knowledge and experience you bring to this conference.

---

*President of the University of Toronto, Toronto, Ontario.

INTRODUCTION TO THE CONFERENCE

J. M. M. DARTE, M.D., F.R.C.P.(C)*

It is nearly 25 years since I first became involved at the Hospital for Sick Children in the treatment of malignant disease in childhood. Hence, it may be interesting to compare the state of affairs at that time with the present.

Like many pediatricians, I was drawn into chemotherapy, which began to burgeon with the folic acid antagonists in 1947; these were applied to the treatment of children with acute leukemia, who, at that time, had an expected survival of about 3.3 months. Wilms' tumor and other childhood malignancies, were considered to have a terrible prognosis. Most centres were reporting overall survivals of less than 30%. We were no exception. Neuroblastoma had an even worse outlook – 14 to 20% survivors. In those days, some patients were allowed to have a spontaneous remission. At that time, in Toronto, we had not a single long-term survivor with medulloblastoma. Children's malignancy was considered just short of a death sentence.

Hodgkin's disease, lymphosarcoma, osteogenic sarcoma, Ewing's and other sarcomas, all had a gloomy outlook.

True, some centres were beginning to report good results in some diseases, such as the Manchester and other English centres' reports of radiotherapy of the whole central nervous system in children with medulloblastoma; and Gross' reports from Boston concerning his results.

It was an era of empiricism and individuality. People like Skipper were providing animal model systems but their voices were not really heard. That era was followed by one of co-operation, of giant strides, both in our understanding of the process of cancer, of the natural history of diseases with which we dealt, and of the nature of the drugs we used.

Perhaps in no other field of malignancy has progress been made so rapidly as in the cancers of childhood. We have now reached the point where Sir Bodley Scott can say: "It is now respectable to talk about 'cure' when discussing leukemia." Throughout the chemotherapeutic world the word "cure" is no longer a dirty word when discussing a leukemic patient; this change in attitude came spontaneously in several centres at about the same time. The outlook in Wilms' tumor was already clearly improving rapidly. Children's cancer, which had been considered to have among the worst of prognoses, now is considered to be among the best – with, of course, some exceptions.

---

*Professor and Chairman, Department of Pediatrics, Memorial University of Newfoundland, St. John's, Newfoundland.

SOME STATISTICS ON CHILDHOOD CANCER IN ONTARIO

A. H. SELLERS, C.D., M.D., D.P.H.*, E. N. MacKAY, M.D., C.M., D.P.H.**
and E. E. McLERIE, B.Sc.†

MORTALITY

Cancer ranks second as a cause of death for both sexes at ages 1-19 years. At ages 1-4 years, it ranks third to accidents and congenital anomalies; at ages 5-9, 10-14 and 15-19 years, it is second only to accidents. The average number of cancer deaths per year at these ages in Ontario during the five years 1965-1969 was about 200: under one year of age – 8; at ages 1-4 – 60 deaths; at ages 5-9 – 57 deaths; at 10-14 – 40 deaths; and at 15-19 – 44 deaths (Table I).

TABLE I

Childhood Cancer by Age and Sex
Ontario, 1965 – 1969

Age Group	Males			Females		
	Deaths	Rate*	Per Cent All Deaths	Deaths	Rate*	Per Cent All Deaths
Under 1	17	4.9	0.2	23	7.0	0.4
1 - 4	170	11.3	13.2	125	8.7	12.1
5 - 9	156	7.8	15.0	128	6.7	18.4
10 - 14	126	6.9	15.0	75	4.3	15.6
15 - 19	144	9.1	7.9	74	4.8	10.4

* Rate per 100,000 population at ages

*Medical Statistician,
**Associate Medical Statistician and
†Statistician, The Ontario Cancer Treatment and Research Foundation, Toronto.

At ages under one year, cancer is relatively unimportant as a cause of death (0.3%). During the years 1965 to 1969, among males: at ages 1-4, cancer contributed 13.2% of all deaths; at ages 5-9 and ages 10-14, 15.0%; and at ages 15-19, 7.9%. The corresponding figures for females were: 12.1%, 18.4%, 15.6% and 10.4%. From 5 to 14 years of age, one death in every six is due to cancer; at ages 1-4, one death in eight is a cancer death.

AGE AND SEX VARIATIONS

The specific cancer mortality rate for this age group (0-19) was 8.4 for males and 6.1 for females per 100,000 population. The age-specific death rate is highest at ages 1-4 for both sexes; followed in males by the age groups 15-19, 5-9, 10-14 and under one year, and in females by the age groups under 1, 5-9, 15-19 and 10-14 years. These differences are also associated with differences in cancer site distribution.

There is a male excess in cancer mortality in each age group except under one year (0.7); the sex ratios of the cancer death rates in the four succeeding age groups are 1.3, 1.2, 1.6 and 1.9 to 1.

PRINCIPAL CANCER SITES

The principal lethal cancer site groups vary with age and sex but, at ages under 20 years, they are: leukemia, brain and other parts of nervous system, Hodgkin's disease and other lymphatic and hematopoietic tissues, and bone and connective tissue (Table II). Leukemia ranks first in all five-year age groups under 20 years, with brain and other nervous system second. (The International Classification of Diseases is as yet unsatisfactory for the classification of childhood neoplasms.)

TABLE II

Childhood Cancer by Site and Sex
Ontario, 1965 – 1969

Site	Males			Females		
	Deaths	Per Cent	Rate*	Deaths	Per Cent	Rate*
Leukaemia & aleukaemia	276	45.0	3.8	203	47.8	2.9
Brain & other nervous system	118	19.3	1.6	84	19.8	1.2
Other lymph & haem. tissue	71	11.6	1.0	27	6.4	0.4
Bone & connective tissue	48	7.8	0.7	36	8.4	0.5
Residual	100	16.3	1.4	75	17.6	1.1
Total	613	100.0	8.4	425	100.0	6.1

* Per 100,000 population ages 0 - 19 years

There is a male excess in cancer mortality at ages 0-19 years in each broad site-group. The sex ratios during 1965-1969 were, for leukemia – 1.3 to 1, brain and other nervous system – 1.4 to 1, Hodgkin's disease and other lymphomas – 2.5 to 1, and bone and connective tissue – 1.4 to 1. This male excess is evident in virtually all childhood age-groups.

TRENDS IN MORTALITY

Cancer has become a relatively more important cause of death among children during the past 20 years; the proportion of deaths from all causes which are attributed to cancer at ages under 20 years has doubled: from 2.5% to 5.0%; at ages 1-19, the proportion has increased from 8.3% to 12.0% for males and from 9.4% to 13.8% for females. These changes are due largely to the reduction in infant mortality, and to the reduction in causes of death other than cancer.

The trend in cancer mortality and in mortality from all causes combined for the age group 1-19 years by sex for the years 1940 to 1970 is illustrated in Fig. 1. Over this 30-year period there has been little noteworthy change in the

TRENDS IN MORTALITY, ALL CAUSES AND CANCER
AGES 1-19
ONTARIO, 1940-70

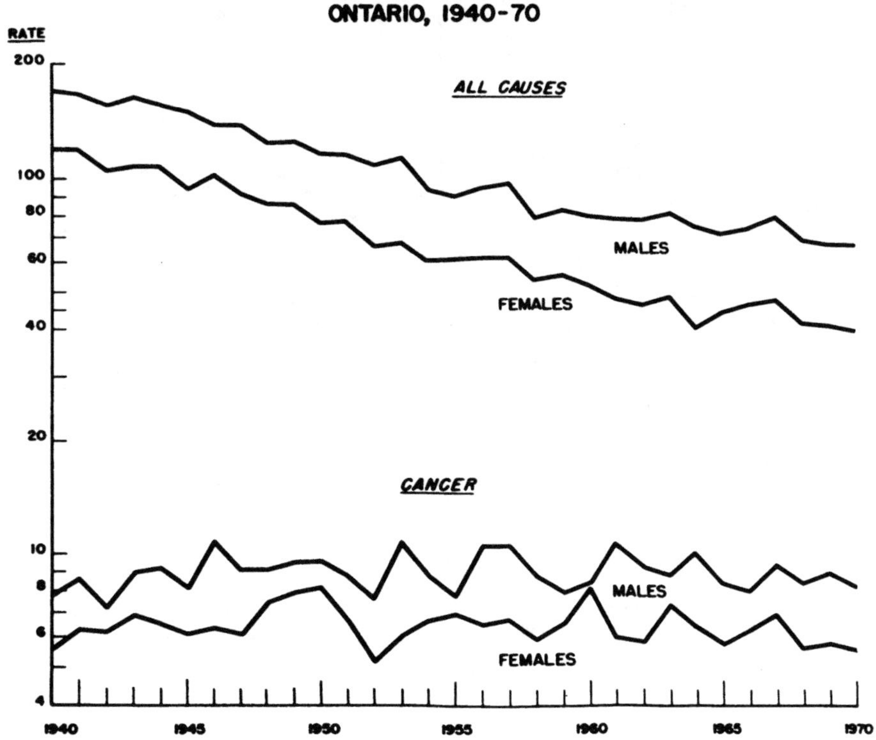

Fig. 1

childhood cancer death rate, except *possibly* a slight decline over the last 10 years. In contrast, the death rate from all causes at ages 1-19 years has declined by about two-thirds for both sexes – from 171 to 67 per 100,000 for males, and from 120 to 40 for females.

TRENDS BY AGE GROUP

Most of the reduction in general mortality during childhood has occurred at ages 1-14 years. The trend in childhood cancer mortality by age-group and sex in five-year periods over the past 20 years, is quite irregular and shows no significant changes (Fig. 2).

CHILDHOOD CANCER MORTALITY BY AGE GROUP AND SEX ONTARIO, 1950-1969

(RATE PER 100,000 POPULATION)

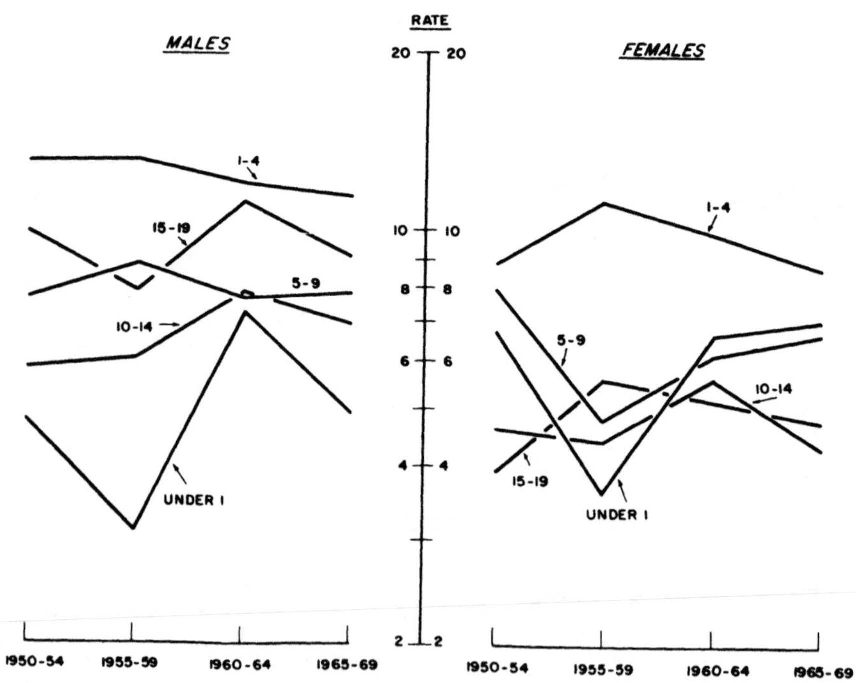

Fig. 2

TRENDS BY CANCER SITE

There is little noteworthy change in the broad site distribution of childhood cancer deaths over the period 1950-54 to 1965-69, except possibly a very slightly favourable trend for the Hodgkin's disease and other lymphoma group (Fig. 3). It is of interest too that there has been a perceptible decline since 1960 in mortality from cancer of the kidney in the age group 0-4 years. A similar reduction has been noted in the United States.

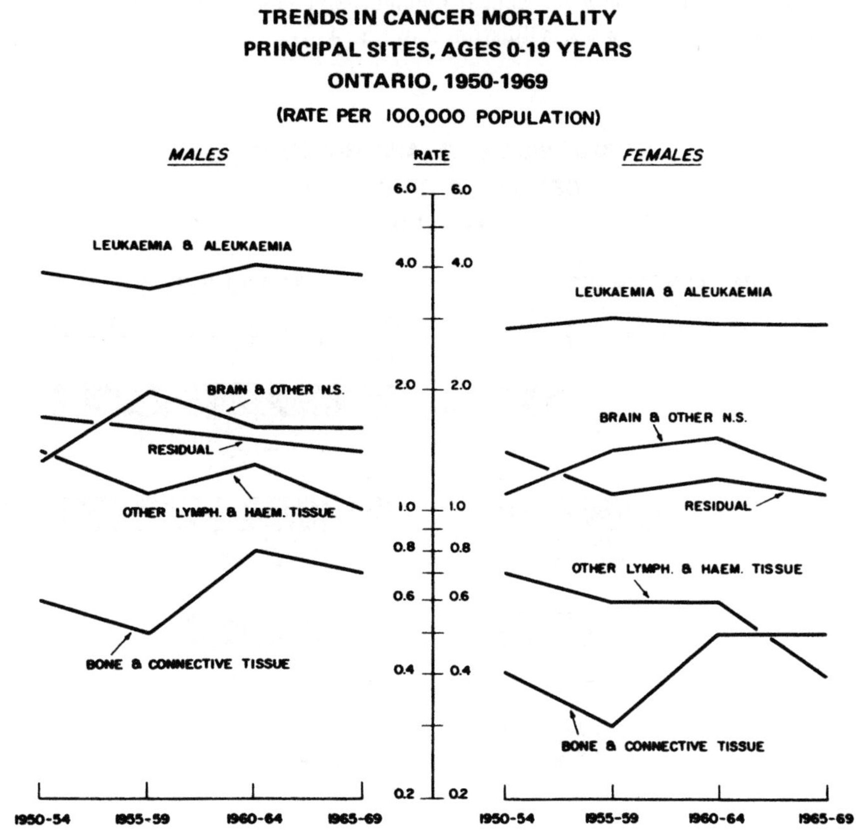

Fig. 3

INCIDENCE

The Ontario Cancer Incidence Survey of 1964-1966 provides reasonably solid information on cancer incidence in Ontario. In 1966 the survey identified 230 new cancer cases among males and 189 new cancer cases among females at ages 0-19 years – rates of 16.0 and 13.8 per 100,000 population respectively. The age-specific incidence rates for *males* exceeded those for females in all age groups under 15 years but, at 15-19 years, there was an excess *female* incidence (in contrast to mortality) due largely to skin cancer (both malignant melanoma and other) and leukemia.

The relationship between cancer incidence and cancer mortality in the age groups under 19 years by sex is illustrated in Fig. 4.

CANCER INCIDENCE AND MORTALITY
AGES UNDER 20 BY SEX
ONTARIO

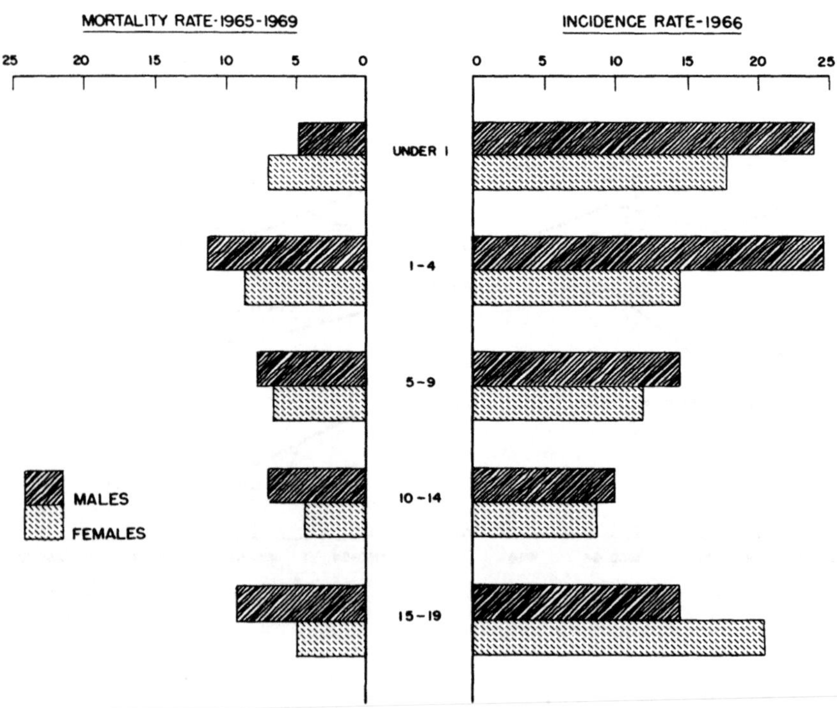

Fig. 4

INTERNATIONAL VARIATIONS

As in adult cancer, there is much variation in childhood cancer mortality throughout the world. Standardized death rates by sex for 10 countries are presented in Fig. 5[1]. Variations in recorded incidence similar to those shown for mortality are evident in the international data published in "Cancer in Five Continents"[2].

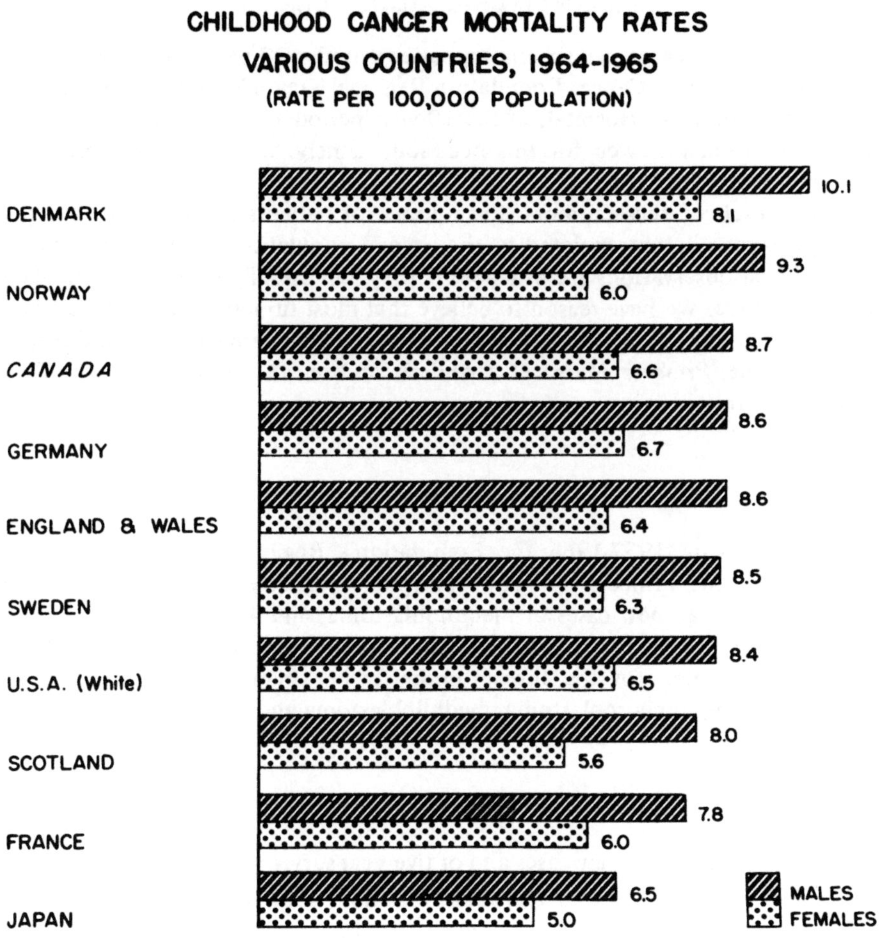

Fig. 5

INCIDENCE AND CASELOAD

In 1971, 156 cancer cases at ages 0-14 years (93 males and 63 females) were first registered at the Regional Cancer Treatment Centres, two-thirds of them at the Princess Margaret Hospital. The estimated number of new cases of cancer at ages 0-14 years in Ontario during the year 1971 was 316; 187 males and 129 females. This indicates that about 50% of the cancer cases in these age groups are registered at a Foundation treatment centre or at the Princess Margaret Hospital.

SELECTED CHILDHOOD TUMORS

From all new cases of cancer among patients under 20 years of age who were registered at Ontario Cancer Foundation Regional Treatment Centres other than the Princess Margaret Hospital, in the 10-year period 1957 through 1966, three types have been reviewed for this occasion, namely, neurcblastoma, medulloblastoma, and Wilms' tumor.

For each of these tumors, the number of patients is very small, and the findings cannot be extrapolated to the general population. Tables summarizing the principal observations are available if they can usefully supplement the data from elsewhere. We have reason to believe that most tumors of these three types that occur in Ontario are seen at the Foundation's Regional Treatment Centres, including the Princess Margaret Hospital, and/or at the Hospital for Sick Children, Toronto.

THE REVIEW GROUPS

During the years 1957-1966 the Foundation's Regional Treatment Centres, other than the Princess Margaret Hospital, registered: 41 new cases of neuroblastoma, 24 new cases of medulloblastoma, and 49 patients with Wilms' tumor at ages under 20 years. In this discussion, the data is examined according to age, stage, etc., for the three tumors, rather than grouping together all material relating to neuroblastoma, medulloblastoma and Wilms' tumor.

AGE

The age distribution of new cases and of five-year survivors are presented in Fig. 6.

Most of the 41 cases of *neuroblastoma* were under five years of age and 18 (all boys) were under two years of age at the first treatment (two cases were in newborn infants). Five of the 18 survived for at least five years without disease, four of these were free of disease at last follow-up and one had metastases by his seventh anniversary. The median survival time after treatment at ages under two years was three months. There were no five-year survivors among the 23 patients (eight girls), who were aged 2 to 16 years at initial treatment; the median survival time was six months. Two cases, included in the present series, were diagnosed as ganglioneuroblastoma. One 17-month-old boy with a spinal tumor was alive and well at five years and beyond; the other, a 14-year-old boy with thoracic and extradural disease at initial treatment, died 10 months later.

The 24 cases of *medulloblastoma* were more evenly spaced over the childhood years. Of these 24 children, seven lived for five years or more after first treatment; six were alive and well at last follow-up, while the seventh was recorded as having residual disease or sequelae throughout his eight or more years of survival. The five-year survivors included one of the 15 boys and six of the nine girls in the series.

All but four of the 49 patients with *Wilms' tumor* were among children under seven years of age, with a peak at ages 2 and 3; the five-year survivors were distributed through all ages. Twenty children (seven of 26 boys and 13 of 23 girls) were alive and well at last follow-up five to 14 years after beginning treatment.

The median ages at initial treatment were: for neuroblastoma two years, for medulloblastoma seven years, and for Wilms' tumor three years.

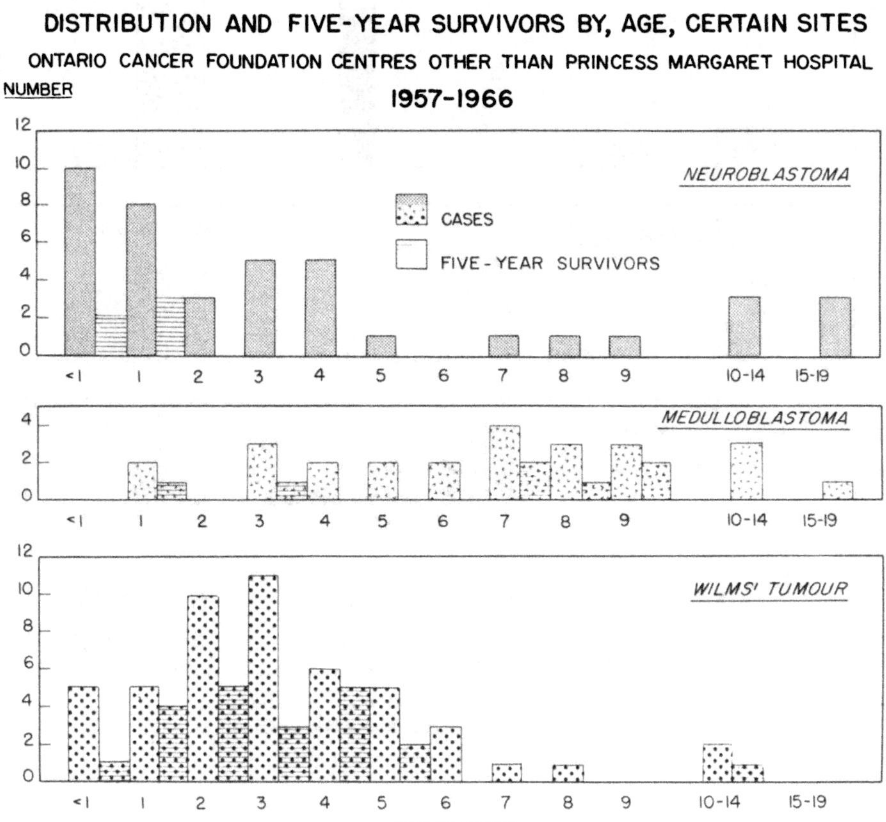

Fig. 6

STAGE OF DISEASE

The source material used for this review was incomplete in respect of anatomical extent of disease; although a fair proportion of cases were "staged", the anatomical extent of disease at treatment was usually not well defined.

The distribution of new cases and five-year survivors by stage is given in Fig. 7. Localized cases do best regardless of treatment; cases with limited local spread can be salvaged but very few with advanced spread (distant metastases) initially survived.

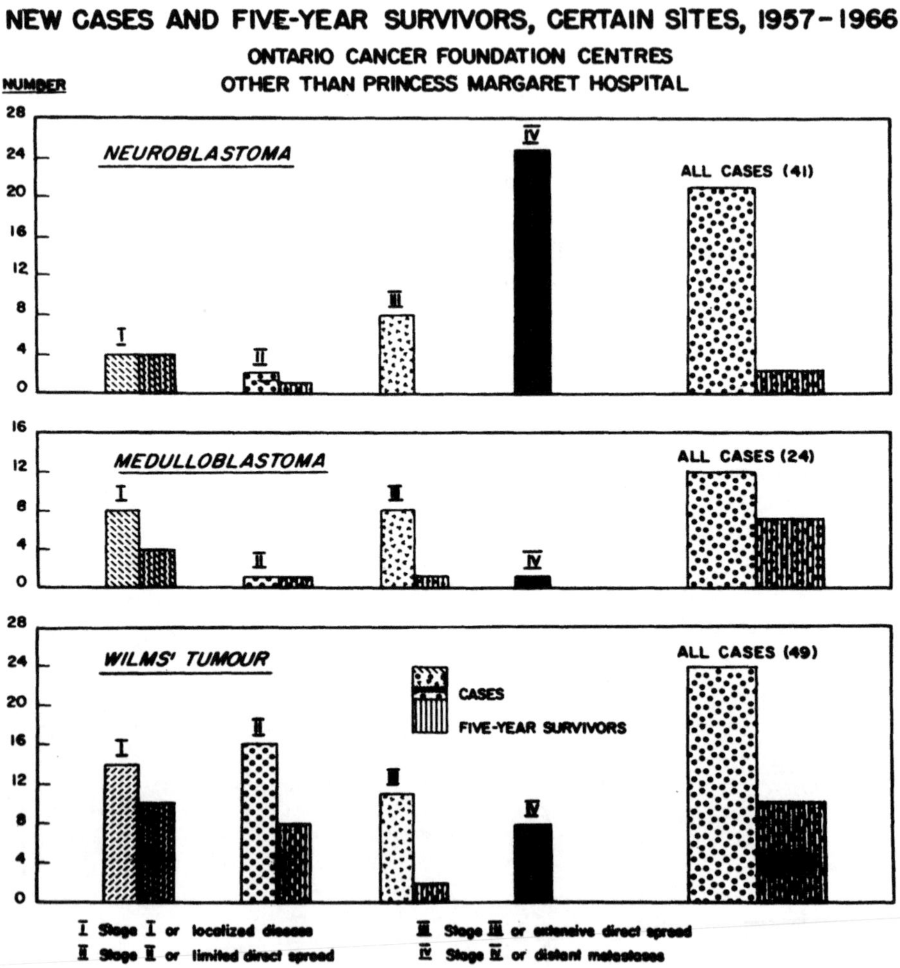

Fig. 7

For *neuroblastoma,* 25 of 41 cases had distant metastases at initial treatment, four had apparently localized disease, two had limited direct spread, and eight had extensive direct spread. (In 10 cases, extent was not stated.) All four cases with apparently localized disease (Stage I) and one of two cases with direct spread (Stage II) survived five years. This last patient had had extension of disease to the great vessels in the chest at the time of initial treatment.

The primary site of the neuroblastoma was not always identified. For 15 children, the adrenal gland appeared to be the primary site; all but one of the 15 had metastases or direct spread on admission, and none lived for more than 17 months. One of 10 children with primary retroperitoneal involvement, and one of five with mediastinal disease, survived five years or more. Three children with spinal or extradural primaries (one of whom had questionable mediastinal involvement), also survived. None of eight children with other or disseminated disease lived as much as two years.

Six children with Stage III disease or distant metastases at initial treatment apparently had remissions lasting from one to 26 months, but died one to 15 months later from recurrence. The median duration of remission was five months, and the median survival after recurrence was 4.5 months.

The chief recorded sites of metastasis on admission to the centres were bone (17 cases), lymph nodes (14 cases), and liver (12 cases). In this small series, there was no evidence that bone involvement carried a poorer prognosis than other metastases.

For *medulloblastoma,* eight of the 24 cases were apparently localized (Stage I), one had limited direct spread (Stage II), eight had extensive direct spread (Stage III), and one had distant metastases at initial treatment. (In six cases, extent was not indicated.) Of the seven five-year survivors, four were Stage I, one each were Stages II and III, and in one the stage was not stated.

For *Wilms' tumor,* 14 of the 49 cases were localized (Stage I), 16 had limited direct spread (Stage II), 11 had extensive direct spread (Stage III), and eight had distant metastases (Stage IV). Of the 20 five-year survivors, 10 were Stage I, eight were Stage II and two were Stage III. Four children with *subsequent* involvement of chest or lung were well five or more years after this involvement.

SURVIVAL

The survival curves of patients with the three types of tumors are presented in Fig. 8. The early mortality is very high for neuroblastoma, and higher for Wilms' tumor than for medulloblastoma (children dying soon after operation for medulloblastoma would not be referred to the treatment centres, so this picture may be biased).

For the 41 cases of *neuroblastoma,* the crude survival rates at the anniversary of beginning treatment were: at one year, 24.4% (10 cases); at two years, 17.1% (seven cases); at three, four and five years, 12.2% (five cases).

For the 24 cases of *medulloblastoma,* the crude survival rates at the anniversary of beginning treatment were: at one year, 70.8% (17 cases); at two years, 45.8% (11 cases); at three years, 37.5% (nine cases), and at four and five years, 29.2% (seven cases). (One child, alive and well without recurrence at the third anniversary, moved to another province and is untraced.)

For the 49 cases of *Wilms' tumor,* the crude survival rates at the anniversary of beginning treatment were: at one year, 63.3% (31 cases); at two years, 49.0% (24 cases); at three years, 44.9% (22 cases); at four years, 42.9% (21 cases), and at five years, 40.8% (20 cases). Of the 20 five-year survivors all were alive and well at last follow-up at five to 14 years after beginning treatment. One child without recurrence died three years after treatment, and one four years after treatment, both from injuries received in motor-vehicle accidents.

For all three tumors, the two-year survival rate is a fair index and the three-year survival rate a very good index of outcome at 5+ years.

Only one child who lived longer than age at onset + 9 months failed to survive at least five years. He had medulloblastoma of the brain extending to the cervical spinal cord, and had been in an institution for many months before his death 46 months after treatment.

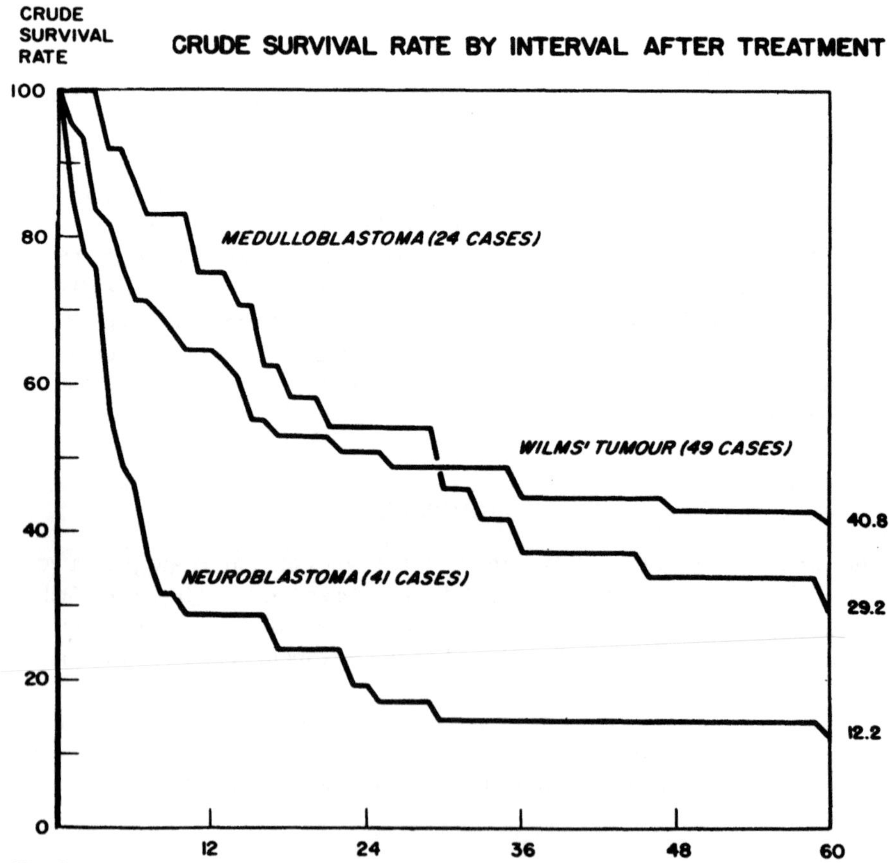

Fig. 8

TREATMENT

Neuroblastoma (41)

Treatment was varied, but all but two children in this group had radiotherapy. The longest median survival time, 26 months, was seen among eight children treated by surgery and radiotherapy; three of the eight lived five years or more. Three children treated by surgery, radiotherapy and chemotherapy lived for three months, 10 months, and more than five years. Fourteen children treated by radiotherapy and chemotherapy (usually cyclophosphamide, but also vincristine, nitrogen mustard, and chlorambucil) had a median survival time of six months, ranging from one to 30 months.

Medulloblastoma (24)

Among 16 children who were treated initially by operation and radiotherapy to both skull and spine, six lived for five years or more; and six children who eventually died from the disease appeared to have remissions lasting from four to 20 months. One 16-year-old boy with Stage IV disease on admission had further radiotherapy at four months for a brain recurrence, and seems to have had a remission of up to 26 months before developing generalized central-nervous-system metastases and dying.

Wilms' Tumor (49)

One of three patients treated by surgery alone, a five-year-old boy with a Stage I tumor, lived for at least 10 years after surgery. Ten of 30 children treated by *radiotherapy and surgery* survived without disease for five years or more (Fig. 9), while nine of 14 children treated by *surgery, radiotherapy and chemotherapy* did so (Fig. 10). With such small numbers, this doubling of the five-year survival rate among children who received adjunctive chemotherapy may not be statistically significant. However, it is interesting to note that, among patients with Stage II or III disease or local spread, seven of nine patients who received surgery, radiotherapy and chemotherapy survived five years, in contrast to only three of 16 who had surgery and radiotherapy but no chemotherapy. (The survivors included two who had nitrogen mustard, one who had cyclophosphamide and cortisone, and four who had actinomycin-D.) this apparent *increase in the salvage of non-localized cases,* together with the increase in median survival time – from 13 to 14 months after surgery alone or with radiotherapy, to more than five years for these modalities *plus* chemotherapy, suggests that chemotherapy does limit disease that cannot be extirpated. Because the chemotherapy was given relatively late in the series, changes in radiotherapy and/or surgical approach may also have contributed to this increase in median survival.

With neuroblastoma and medulloblastoma, all patients in the present series who had *recurrences* died of cancer. With Wilms' tumor, this was not so. Four children with disease thought to be localized or in Stage II, were initially treated with surgery, radiotherapy, and actinomycin–D, or nitrogen mustard at operation; they developed lung or chest metastases three to nine months later, were variously treated, and were all alive and well at least five years after the recurrence. (One child had cobalt-60 for the recurrence; one deep x-ray and cortisone; one lobectomy and cyclophosphamide for two years; and one cobalt-60, actinomycin-D, and lobectomy.) Four other children, three of whom had Stage III disease, were initially treated by nephrectomy and cobalt-60: they developed chest or lung metastases six weeks to perhaps a year later, and subsequently died. Seven children with recurrences in areas other than the lung or chest also failed to survive. The median survival after recurrence for 15 patients was 13 months, compared with the interval of only five months between initial treatment and recurrence.

WILMS' TUMOR-SURVIVAL AFTER FIRST TREATMENT, BY EXTENT OF DISEASE AND INITIAL AND SUBSEQUENT TREATMENT METHOD, 1957-1966

ONTARIO CANCER FOUNDATION CENTRES OTHER THAN PRINCESS MARGARET HOSPITAL

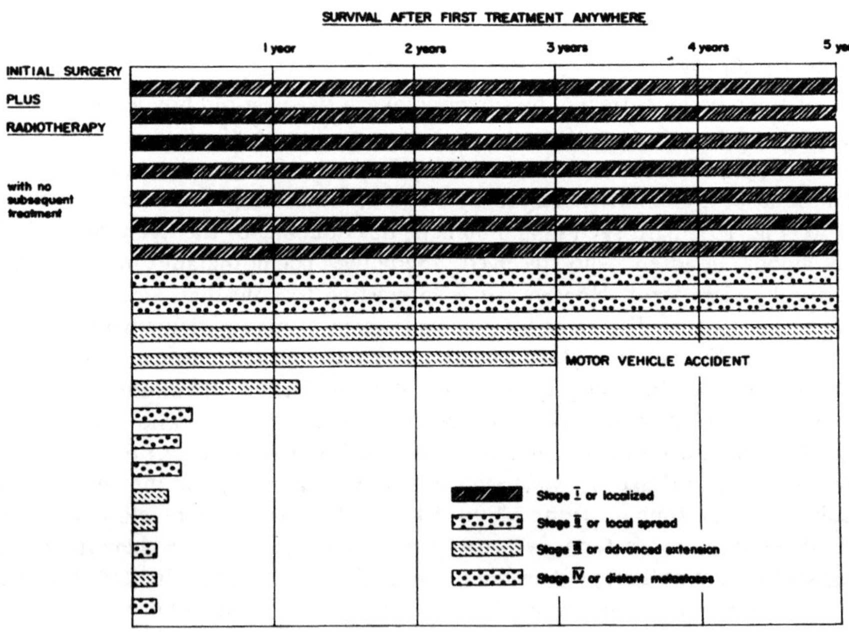

Fig. 9

WILMS' TUMOR-SURVIVAL AFTER FIRST TREATMENT, BY EXTENT OF DISEASE AND INITIAL AND SUBSEQUENT TREATMENT METHOD, 1957-1966

ONTARIO CANCER FOUNDATION CENTRES OTHER THAN PRINCESS MARGARET HOSPITAL

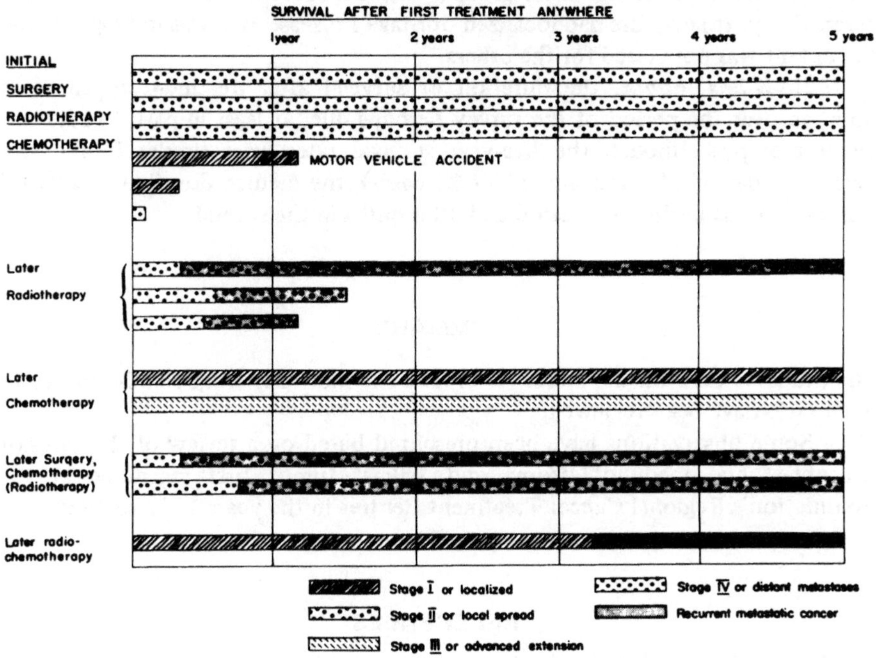

Fig. 10

CHANGES IN SURVIVAL

For *neuroblastoma* there appeared to be little change in survival over the period of the review: the median survival time for 16 children registered in 1957-1961 was four months, and for the 25 children in 1962-1966 it was six months (Table III).

TABLE III

Changes in Survival, 1957 - 61, 1962 - 66 – Certain Sites
Ontario Cancer Foundation Centres Other Than Princess Margaret Hospital

	Neuroblastoma		Medulloblastoma		Wilms' Tumour	
	1957 - 61	1962 - 66	1957 - 61	1962 - 66	1957 - 61	1962 - 66
Cases registered	16	25	8	16	25	24
Alive at 5 years	2	3	–	7	9	11
Median survival time	4 mos.	6 mos.	9 mos.	36 mos.	14 mos.	48 mos.

The outlook for *medulloblastoma* did appear to improve over the review period, and to be related to irradiation of both skull and spine. None of the eight children registered in the years 1957-1961 survived five years, but seven of the 16 registered in 1962-1966 did so. The median survival time for the earlier group was nine months; for the latter group it was 36 months. However, four of the seven five-year survivors had localized or Stage I disease, one was in Stage II, and the extent was not stated for the others.

In *Wilms' tumor,* the duration of survival after treatment appeared to improve over the period of the survey perhaps due, at least in part, to adjuvant chemotherapy; although the five-year survival rates were similar in the two periods (nine of 25 cases and 11 of 24 cases), the median duration of survival was 14 months in the first period and 48 months in the second.

SUMMARY

The available data on the incidence of, and the mortality from childhood cancer in Ontario have been reviewed.

Some observations have been presented based on a review of the cases of neuroblastoma, medulloblastoma and Wilms' tumor first registered at the Foundation's Regional Cancer Treatment Centres in the years 1957 to 1966.

REFERENCES

1 SEGI, M.: Cancer Mortality for Selected Sites in 24 Countries, No. 5 (1964-1965), Department of Public Health, Tohoku University School of Medicine, Sendai, Japan, August 1969.

2 DOLL, R., MUIR, C. and WATERHOUSE, J.: Cancer Incidence in Five Continents, Volume II, 1970, distributed for the International Union Against Cancer by Springer – Verlag, Berlin – Heidelberg – New York.

THE MANCHESTER CHILDREN'S TUMOR REGISTRY

P. H. MORRIS JONES*

The Manchester Children's Tumor Registry was established in September 1953 to collect data on the true incidence of malignant disease in children and to define the therapeutic problems which had to be faced: e.g., exactly how many children died, and what could be done to reduce this mortality.

Children were included in the registry only if they were under the age of 15 years and were living in the Manchester region at the time of diagnosis. The region has a population of five million: one million of these are children. The region covers an area varying from industrialized cotton towns to the Lake District and the rich farming area of Cheshire. In numbers and race the population has remained stable over the last 30 years.

The value of the figures produced in a registry depends on the accuracy and the completeness of the information about each patient. It was decided at the outset that it was impossible to devise a form containing all the questions which might be relevant to the disease. Hence, photostat copies of the hospital notes or full summaries made by qualified medical staff employed by the Registry have formed the basis of an ongoing record of each patient. In retrospect this method has been accurate with regard to clinical data but leaves big gaps in the epidemiological information, which is difficult to obtain retrospectively without distress to the parents.

Our definition of the "date of diagnosis" is that date on which the child was first seen by a consultant, for this is known for almost all children. This date is used as the reference time for all data analysis.

In every case with a tissue diagnosis, the sections have been reviewed by a panel of pathologists drawn from centres in the United Kingdom, the United States of America and in this city, and the final diagnoses have been based on their reports and the clinical findings.

We have now collated data from a 15-year period and this material will now be discussed. Table I breaks down into major categories the 1583 cases in the Registry. Maximum follow-up is now approaching 19 years and the minimum is four years. The overall survival, 31%, will, of course, fall further because of the fall off in leukemic patients and in those with gliomas. Table II demonstrates a representative year's caseload and shows that these figures can be taken as percentages because the average incidence for each year is 100 cases. Over the years there has been no demonstrable increase and this is confirmed by the national death-rate figures. Table III shows that in the group as a whole there is a sex difference in cancer incidence.

---

*Lecturer in Pediatric Oncology, The Department of Child Health, University of Manchester and Children's Hospital, Manchester.

TABLE I

Manchester Children's Tumor Registry
Cases Included 1954-1968 (Assessed 1972)

Category	Alive	Dead	Total
Leukemias	11	454	465
Non-leukemic reticuloendothelial	58	88	146
Gliomas	90	193	283
Sympathetic	25	90	115
Retinoblastomas	43	8	51
Connective tissue	90	101	191
Renal	28	59	87
Gonadal	8	6	14
Teratomas	34	16	50
Epithelial	38	25	63
Ewing's	2	26	28
Rare miscellaneous	30	18	48
Third ventricular (clinical diagnosis only)	6	4	10
Unclassified	3	29	32
Total	466	1117	1583

TABLE II

Manchester Children's Tumor Registry
Average Annual Incidence of Tumors in Children
(Population under 15 years – 1 million)

Leukemia	29
Non-leukemic reticuloendothelial	9
Gliomas	17
Sympathetic nervous system tumors	8
Retinoblastomas	3
Connective tissue tumors	12
Wilms' tumors	5
Other nephrogenital ridge tumors	1
Teratomas	4
Epithelial tumors	4
Ewing's tumors	2
Miscellaneous tumors	4
Malignant unclassified tumors	2
Total	100

TABLE III

Sex Differences

Category	Males	Females
Leukemias	253	212
Lymphosarcomas	32	13
Hodgkin's disease	31	16
Medulloblastomas	54	20
Neuroblastomas	67	35
Embryonic sarcomas	39	27
Other connective tissue tumors	71	54
Presacral teratomas	3	11
Others	329	316
Total	879	704

If we now look at the subgroups in more detail, the pattern comes through more clearly. There were 465 leukemias (Table IV). Of these, 125 were labelled "stem cell", a diagnosis that was made at the outset. The validity of this is borne out by the fact that this group did not survive as long as the definite acute lymphocytic leukemia (ALL) group. The difference in survival by age is partly accounted for by the fact that fewer younger children were referred to the centre.

TABLE IV

Manchester Children's Tumor Registry
Leukemia, 1954-1968

Acute lymphoblastic	251
Acute stem cell	125
Acute myeloid	60
Acute monocytic	14
Acute myelomonocytic	9
Acute erythroleukemia	2
Chronic myeloid	4
Total	465

Until I began to work full time in Children's Hospital in the care of these children, less than one-half of them were referred to our centre in the University of Manchester. Even then, we recognized a significant difference in the survival depending on whether these children were treated in the centre. Now I treat some 95% of them and survival has improved even further, because of increased experience, and the superior facilities available in the Children's Hospital.

If we refer again to Table I we are reminded of the overall distribution of these tumors and the proportion of solid reticuloendothelial tumors. In the lymphosarcoma group, all our survivors either had neck or inguinal nodes, or gastrointestinal tract primaries.

The central nervous system (CNS) tumors have been divided into histological types (Table V). Our data shows 58% of all these tumors occur in 3% of the brain volume, namely midline structures including the cerebellar vermis. This finding seems to suggest that the cause of gliomas in childhood operates in early fetal life.

TABLE V

Manchester Children's Tumor Registry
Gliomas, 1954-1968 (Assessed 1972)

Category	Alive	Dead	Total
Astrocytomas	57	71	128
Medulloblastomas	16	58	74
Ependymomas	7	33	40
Oligodendrogliomas	1	4	5
Astroblastomas	–	1	1
Gliomas (type unspecified)	–	5	5
Clinical diagnosis only	9	21	30
Total	90	193	283

The 51 retinoblastomas in the register (Table VI) are divided into the bilateral and unilateral cases. Seventeen children in five families inherited the disease. Two families had two affected children.

The neuroblastomas present an unhappy picture. Our overall results are as depressing as those of any other published series; when broken down, they vary from a 73% survival in the Stage I cases to a single survivor in Stage IV.

Renal tumors are, of course, mostly nephroblastomas; the survival of children with these tumors is most unsatisfactory in comparison with those in selected series. However, in recent years we can demonstrate that there is a difference in survival – 60% compared to 30%, depending on whether the children are treated in the Children's Hospital or elsewhere. This further strengthens our recommendation that treatment for cancer in childhood be centralized.

The other subgroups are tabulated in Tables VI to XI, namely, connective tissue tumors, gonadal tumors, teratomas, epithelial tumors and the rare group.

TABLE VI

Manchester Children's Tumor Registry
Retinoblastoma, 1954-1968 (Assessed 1972)

Alive		Dead	
Unilateral	Bilateral	Unilateral	Bilateral
23	20	4	4

TABLE VII

Manchester Children's Tumor Registry
Connective Tissue, 1954-1968 (Assessed 1972)

Category	Alive	Dead	Total
Embryonic sarcomas	12	54	66
Fibromatous tumors	41	7	48
Osteo- and chondrosarcomas	6	28	34
Synoviomas	5	8	13
Lipomatous tumors	8	2	10
Osteoid osteomas	7	–	7
Osteoclastomas	5	–	5
Mesenchymomas	–	2	2
Leiomyosarcomas	1	–	1
Chondroblastomas	1	–	1
Myxomas	1	–	1
Osteomas	1	–	1
Uncertain	2	–	2
Total	90	101	191

TABLE VIII

Manchester Children's Tumor Registry
Gonadal, 1954-1968 (Assessed 1972)

Category	Alive	Dead	Total
Orchioblastomas	2	1	3
Endodermal sinus tumors	–	3	3
Granulosa-theca cell tumors	2	–	2
Arrhenoblastomas	1	–	1
Dysgerminomas	3	–	3
Carcinoma ovary	–	2	2
Total	8	6	14

TABLE IX

Manchester Children's Tumor Registry
Teratomas, 1954-1968 (Assessed 1972)

Category	Alive	Dead	Total
Ovarian	17	1	18
Presacral	7	7	14
Testicular	7	–	7
Chest	1	1	2
Intracranial	–	4	4
Spinal canal	1	–	1
Pelvic	1	–	1
Ovary and lung	–	1	1
Heart	–	1	1
Bladder	–	1	1
Total	34	16	50

TABLE X

Manchester Children's Tumor Registry
Epithelial Tumors, 1954-1968 (Assessed 1972)

Category	Alive	Dead	Total
Salivary glands	9	1	10
Carcinoma – floor of mouth	–	1	1
Pharyngeal lymphoepitheliomas	2	7	9
Ameloblastomas	2	–	2
Thyroid tumors	3	–	3
Parathyroid tumors	1	–	1
Adrenal cortical tumors	2	2	4
Carcinoma – colon	–	2	2
Carcinoma – breast	1	–	1
Tumors of the dermal appendages	2	–	2
Benign calcifying epitheliomas	3	–	3
Craniopharyngiomas	9	8	17
Carcinoma – bronchus	–	2	2
Carcinoma – thymus	–	1	1
Pituitary tumors	1	1	2
Carcinoid (appendix)	3	–	3
Total	38	25	63

TABLE XI

Manchester Children's Tumor Registry
Rare Miscellaneous Tumors, 1954-1968 (Assessed 1972)

Category	Alive	Dead	Total
Tumors of nerve sheath	18	1	19
Pinealomas	–	7	7
Hepatic tumors	–	7	7
Granular myoblastomas	5	–	5
Malignant melanomas	1	1	2
Fibroadenoma breast	1	–	1
Progonoma	1	–	1
Paraganglioma	1	–	1
Chemodectoma	1	–	1
Chordoma	1	–	1
Meningeal melanoma	–	1	1
Islet-cell tumor of pancreas	–	1	1
Scalp tumor of uncertain origin	1	–	1
Total	30	18	48

Returning to Table I, we find that of 1583 children, 1117 have already died. What can we learn from these figures? Are these children diagnosed early enough?

Considering that, on the average, a general practitioner sees only one child with a tumor every 20 years, it is perhaps surprising that they reach hospital so early. A recent analysis showed that there was a delay only in the diagnosis of the CNS tumors and in those of the cervical lymph nodes. The numbers who would have lived by virtue of earlier diagnosis and present therapy must be very small. What is the effect of treatment? Most of the survivors had surgery or a combination of surgery with radiotherapy. Nonetheless, the results are not encouraging. Why do we fail? In the children who died, 72% of the tumors fell into four absolute categories: those that were disseminated at diagnosis; the posterior abdominal wall tumors, which were often incompletely removed; the brainstem and third ventricle tumors, which are difficult surgical problems; and the connective tissue tumors. Therefore, we have to look for earlier methods of diagnosis based on a high index of suspicion associated with very careful epidemiological and genetic evaluation. In the tumors not amenable to complete removal, we must make better use of chemotherapy and radiotherapy so as to enhance the chances of successful resection. The use of immunotherapy in certain selected cases must also be explored.

Because very few children included in this review had any chemotherapy (certainly up to the end of 1968), we hope that they will act as a control group in subsequent comparisons with our present and future cases, most of whom are now on planned chemotherapy programs.

We intend to expand our collection of prospective epidemiological data and to correlate this with similar data from other parts of the world so as to hasten the collection of meaningful series in these important and difficult tumors.

WILMS' TUMOR: A REVIEW OF THE TORONTO EXPERIENCE

M. J. SONLEY, M.D., F.R.C.P.(C)*

Between 1920 and 1968, 211 children with Wilms' tumor had at least part of their primary treatment at the Hospital for Sick Children or the Princess Margaret Hospital. Patients referred after the completion of their primary treatment have been excluded. The diagnosis was confirmed histologically in all cases. All of the children have been followed for at least four years after diagnosis, and 201 have been followed five years or more. There were 113 males and 98 females with a median age of two years (Fig. 1).

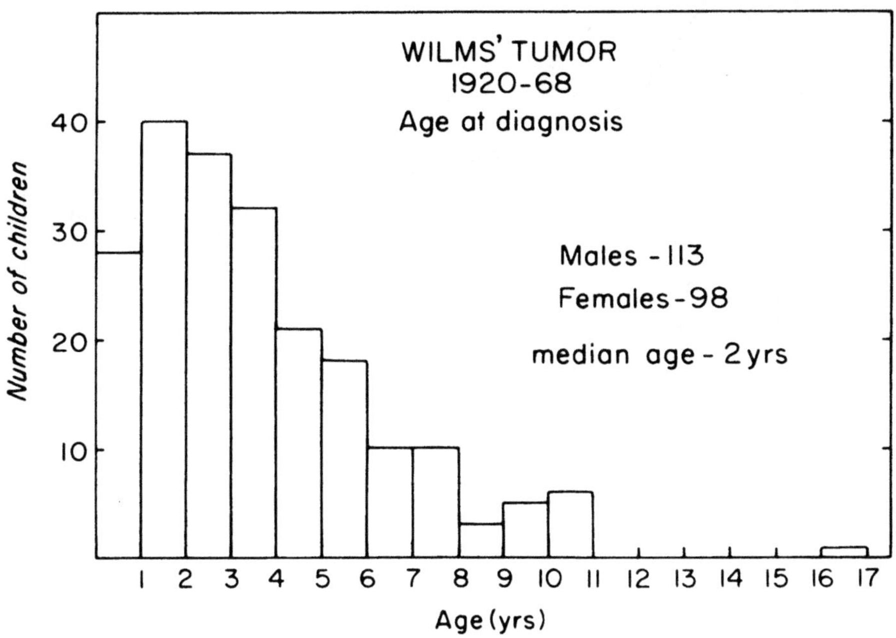

Fig. 1. Wilms' Tumor: Toronto experience 1920-1968, age at diagnosis.

*Chief, Department of Pediatrics, The Princess Margaret Hospital, Toronto; Department of Hematology, The Hospital for Sick Children, Toronto; and Assistant Professor of Pediatrics, University of Toronto.

Any analysis of the results of treatment of Wilms' tumor must take into account the tremendous changes in treatment, which have taken place over the past 50 years, and particularly between 1950 and 1962. Because a major change in the radiotherapy and follow-up can be pinpointed at 1957 when J. M. M. Darte became our first pediatric radiotherapist, the patients have been divided into two groups: those treated before 1957, and those treated since January 1957. Between 1920 and 1956, 95 children were seen with Wilms' tumor and 116 have been treated since 1957.

The improvement in survival during the two periods has been dramatic (Fig. 2). Before 1957, only 23% of the children were alive five years later, compared to 66% since 1957. Since no patient in this series is known to have died of Wilms' tumor more than five years after diagnosis, we consider that 66% of the children treated since 1957 are probably cured.

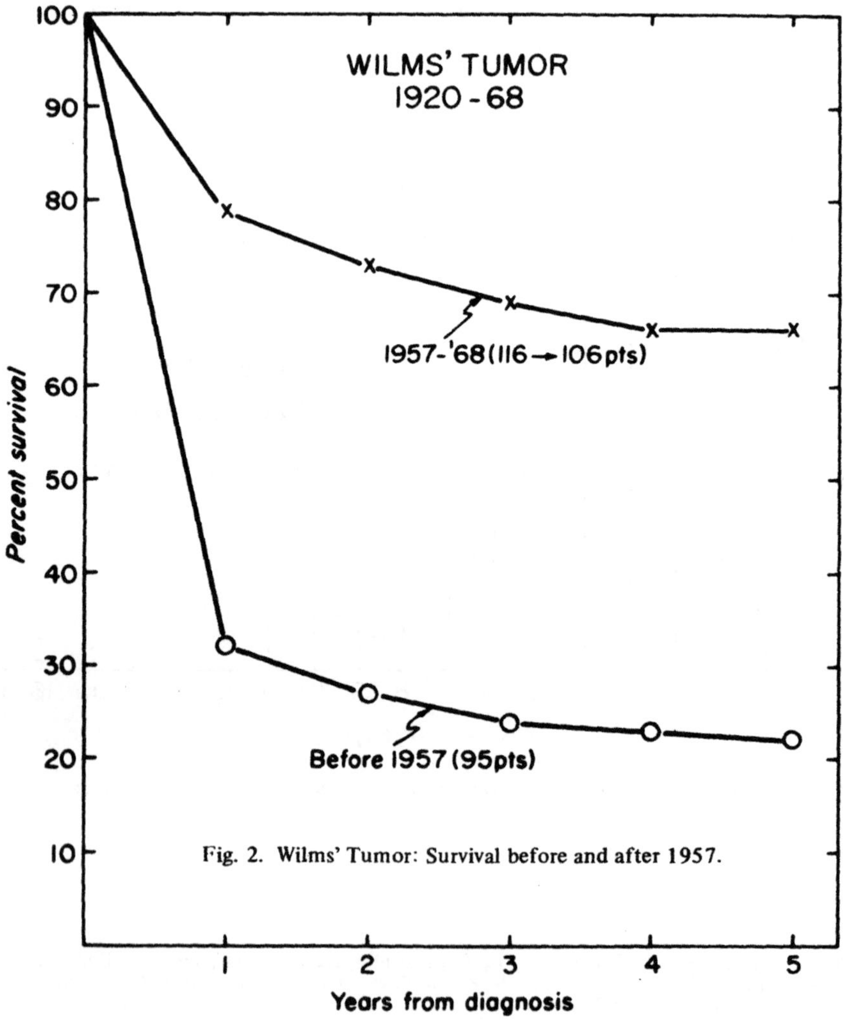

Fig. 2. Wilms' Tumor: Survival before and after 1957.

STAGING

The National Wilms' Tumor Study Committee has subdivided the children with Wilms' tumor into five groups, based on the extent of tumor before starting treatment (Table I). In Group I, the tumor was confined within the kidney and the kidney has been completely resected. In Group II, the tumor extended beyond the kidney, penetrating the capsule or involving the renal vein or hilar nodes, but the kidney and all of the tumor were completely resected. In Group III, some tumor tissue has been left in the abdomen because the tumor ruptured before or during operation, a biopsy was done previously, the para-aortic nodes were infiltrated, or the tumor has been incompletely resected. In Group IV, hematogenous spread to the lung, liver, brain, or bone has already occurred, and in Group V, the tumor is bilateral.

TABLE I

Wilms' Tumor: Clinical Groups*

Group I	– Tumor limited to kidney and completely resected
Group II	– Tumor extends beyond the kidney but is completely resected
Group III	– Residual non-hematogenous tumor confined to abdomen
Group IV	– Hematogenous metastases
Group V	– Bilateral renal involvement either initially or subsequently

*The National Wilms' Tumor Study Committee.

Our cases have been subdivided according to this classification (Table II). Specific negative information is necessary to classify a patient into Group I, e.g., the capsule is *not* penetrated and the renal vein is *not* infiltrated. Determining in retrospect whether a tumor belonged in Group I or Group II is often difficult, particularly in children seen before 1957, because negative data about capsular penetration and involvement of renal vein or renal nodes were rarely noted in the pathology reports. We have placed such children into a combined group (Group I or II) because of inadequate information about the microscopic findings. Since 1957, 63% of the children were either in Group I or Group II (approximately one-third were Group I, one-third Group II and one-third were either I or II). Twenty-four per cent had residual tumor in the abdomen after operation (Group III), 10% had distant metastases at diagnosis (Group IV), and 3% presented with bilateral tumors (Group V). One patient who had bilateral tumors and lung metastases, has been included only in Group IV.

TABLE II

Wilms' Tumor: Distribution of 211 Cases

Group	1920-1956		1957-1968	
		Per cent		Per cent
I	1		24	
II	5	51	20	63
I or II	45		19	
III		39		24
IV		7		10*
V		1		3
Not stated		1		–
		100%		100%

*One case had bilateral tumors as well.

SURVIVAL

Since 1957 the survival has improved in every group (Table III). In Groups I and II, the five-year survival has almost doubled from 40% to 75%; and in Group III, it soared from 5% to 52%. In Group IV, no patient survived for five years before 1957, whereas, since 1957, three of eight patients are alive and well five years after diagnosis, and of the 12 patients who have been followed for four years, six are alive and free of disease. The one patient who had bilateral tumors before 1957 died, but three of the four children treated since 1957 are alive and well five years later. The child with bilateral tumor and lung metastases is also well four years after diagnosis.

Several factors are responsible for this marked improvement. Advances have taken place in all aspects of treatment, including surgery, radiotherapy, chemotherapy, the routine follow-up, and the treatment of pulmonary metastases.

TABLE III

Wilms' Tumor: Five-Year Survival

Group	Before 1957			1957-1968		
	No. of Pts.	Alive (after 5 yr.)	% Alive	No. of Pts.	Alive (after 5 yr.)	% Alive
I + II	49	20	40	68	51	75
III	37	2	5	27	14	52
IV	7	–	–	8	3	(38)*
V	1	–	–	4**	3	(75)

*Four-year survival = 6/12 (50%).
**One patient also included under Group IV.

Surgery

In the early 1950's, the surgical approach changed from a small incision in the loin through which the tumor often had to be removed piecemeal, to a large transverse or vertical abdominal incision, which was occasionally extended to a thoracoabdominal approach for extremely large tumors. Because of the abdominal approach, the renal vein could be tied early in the procedure possibly preventing the spread of tumor cells during manipulation of the kidney. The liver, the other kidney, the para-aortic lymph nodes, and the rest of the abdomen could be palpated and examined visually to determine the total extent of the tumor. In most cases, the tumor could be removed intact through the larger incision. Since 1957, the proportion of patients who have had complete resection of their tumor has doubled, undoubtedly improving survival (Table IV).

TABLE IV

Wilms' Tumor: Treatment

		1920-1956	1957-1968
Surgery:			
Resection	– complete	43	90
	– partial	37	21
	– biopsy	6	2
	– not stated	4	–
No Surgery		5	3
	TOTAL	95	116

Radiotherapy

Before 1957, the radiation field was almost always confined to the tumor bed (Table V). Even when the tumor spilled into the abdominal cavity during operation, or was incompletely resected, only the renal area was radiated. After 1957, the whole abdomen was radiated in almost all children over the age of two years and in those under two who had extension beyond the capsule, spill of the tumor or infiltration of lymph nodes. At that time it was thought that all patients over two years of age had a worse prognosis. In girls, the pelvis was shielded to protect the ovaries unless the tumor had ruptured so, in them. approximately three-fourths of the abdomen was radiated. The tumor dose was 2500 rads in four weeks. When the whole abdomen was radiated, the normal kidney was shielded in the posterior field and received approximately one-half the tumor dose.

It seems likely that a major reason for the poor survival of children in Group III before 1957 was the failure to adequately irradiate all of the tumor, and, that the change in radiotherapy was responsible, at least in part, for the improved survival in Group III since 1957. The effect of the change in radiotherapy cannot be properly evaluated because only a small number of children were treated with the enlarged field before actinomycin-D was added to the regimen. The relative contribution of each to the improved survival cannot be determined.

TABLE V

Wilms' Tumor: Treatment

			Before 1957	1957-1968
Radiotherapy:				
Field	– renal bed		42	21
	– abdomen	whole	–	53
		3/4	–	21
		+ chest	4	9
		+ chest prophylactic	–	3
	– renal bed (+ chest prophylactic)		4	–
	– tumor (pre-op)		7	3
	– other		2	4
No Radiotherapy			36	2

Follow-up

Follow-up of the children before 1957 tended to be inconsistent and irregular. Since 1957 the children have had a physical examination and chest x-ray every month for the first year, every two months for the second year, every three months for the third year, every four months for the fourth year, every six months in the fifth year, and yearly until 10 years after the diagnosis. Thus, metastases have been recognized and treated earlier than they were before 1957.

Treatment of Pulmonary Metastases

Before 1957, metastases to the lungs were often not treated. Only two patients had irradiation of the whole lung and five had a portion of the lung irradiated (Table VI). Since 1957, 28 children have had whole lung irradiation to a tumor dose of 2000 rads in four weeks. Twenty-two of them were given intravenous actinomycin-D in a course of five daily doses of 15 μg./kg./day during the course of radiation. Of the 22 patients treated with pulmonary irradiation and a course of actinomycin-D, 14 (64%) are alive with no evidence of disease four years after their diagnosis. Only one of the eight patients treated with whole-lung irradiation but no chemotherapy, is alive four years after diagnosis. This salvage of at least one-half of the patients who develop pulmonary metastases unquestionably has improved the survival rate.

TABLE VI

Wilms' Tumor: Treatment of Pulmonary Metastases

	1920-1956	1957-1968
XRT to whole lung	2	6
XRT to whole lung + Actinomycin-D	–	22
XRT to partial lung	5	2
Surgery	1	–
Chemotherapy	1	2
Not stated	1	1
Nil	7	–

Actinomycin-D

Actinomycin-D, the last of the major improvements in treatment, has received most of the credit for the increase in survival rate. Unfortunately, no controlled trials have been carried out, and an analysis of its true worth is almost impossible in retrospective studies. The introduction of actinomycin-D meant that chemotherapists and pediatricians became more closely involved in the primary treatment of Wilms' tumor and in the follow-up of these children. It generated renewed interest in the tumor and a more optimistic and aggressive approach to the treatment.

Actinomycin-D was not used in Toronto before 1962. Initially, a course of five consecutive daily injections was given during radiotherapy and no further therapy was given unless the tumor recurred.

It was given only to children over two years of age and to those children under two who had extension of the tumor beyond the kidney. By approximately 1967, the age limit was lowered to one year of age, and some children with tumor extending beyond the kidney were given multiple courses; the first course immediately after operation, and then at six weeks, and 12 weeks postoperatively, and every three months for 18 months (Table VII). A total of 62 children received actinomycin-D during the primary treatment and 15 of these were given multiple courses.

TABLE VII

Wilms' Tumor: Chemotherapy

Actinomycin-D:	Before 1957	1957-1968
Single course	–	47
Multiple courses (18 mo.)	–	15
Other dose schedule	–	2
None	95	52

Actinomycin-D was added to the treatment in the hope that it might eradicate tumor cells beyond the field of radiation. If it has been effective, it should have decreased the incidence of distant metastases. However, when children who had adequate surgery *plus* adequate radiotherapy *plus* actinomycin-D are compared with those who had similar surgery and radiotherapy but no actinomycin-D, the incidence of distant metastases is approximately the same in each group (Table VIII). This table includes children in Groups I to III. If only those in Groups I and II are considered, the incidence of distant metastases is the same whether actinomycin-D was given or not. The number of children in Group III is too small to demonstrate meaningful differences (Table IX). When the four-year survival figures are compared (Table X), survival is less among those who did not receive actinomycin-D, but since the same number of metastases developed in both groups, survival is decreased because those who developed metastases did not do as well when the metastases were treated. If at least 50% of those with lung metastases had survived, as one should expect with current treatment, the survival rate would have been the same.

TABLE VIII

Wilms' Tumor: Influence of Actinomycin-D on Subsequent Metastases Groups I-III

Treatment	Total No. Pts.	Distant Metastases					Local Recurrence
		No. Pts.	Lung	Liver	Bone	Other Kidney	
S + XRT + Act-D	55	24 (44%)	20	2	2	–	3
S + XRT	42	17 (40%)	12	3	–	2*	2

*Likely second primary tumor.

TABLE IX

Wilms' Tumor: Influence of Actinomycin-D on Subsequent Metastases

Treatment	Total No. Pts.	Distant Metastases					Local Recurrence
		No. Pts.	Lung	Liver	Bone	Other Kidney	
Groups I and II:							
S + XRT + Act-D	37	13	10	1	2	–	1
S + XRT – Act-D	35	12	8	2	–	2*	–
Group III:							
S + XRT + Act-D	18	11	10	1	–	–	2
S + XRT – Act-D	7	5	4	1	–	–	2

*Likely second primary tumor.

TABLE X

Wilms' Tumor: Influence of Actinomycin-D on Four-Year Survival

Treatment	All Cases			Patients Treated Since 1957					
				Groups I and II			Group III		
	No. of Pts.	Alive	%	No. of Pts.	Alive	%	No. of Pts.	Alive	%
(S + XRT) + Act-D	55	43	78	37	31	83	18	12	(66)
(S + XRT) – Act-D	42	28	66	35	23	66	7	2	–

With respect to the effect of the age of the patient on these results, one might argue that since, initially, we gave actinomycin-D more frequently to children over two years of age, that group might have more recurrences, and that actinomycin-D had permitted them to do as well as the group who were not primarily given actinomycin-D (the younger children). But, it is not the age that influences prognosis but the group or *stage* of the tumor. When all the cases are considered, children in Group I or Group II who were under two years of age, did no better than older children in Groups I and II. Children less than two years old who are in Group III, do just as badly as children of any age in Group III (Table XI). The reason that the survival rate is better in children under two, is not merely because of their age, but because a greater proportion of children under two are in Groups I and II at the time of diagnosis – (78% compared to 48% for those over two). This may be because Wilms' tumor is discovered earlier in infants because physicians examine them more frequently and their parents handle them more frequently.

TABLE XI

Wilms' Tumor: Influence of Age on Survival
All Patients 1920-1968

Age	Total No. Pts.	Groups I and II		Group III		Group IV		Group V	
		No. Pts.	Alive 4 yr.	No. Pts.	Alive 4 yr.	No. Pts.	Alive	No. Pts.	Alive
<2 yr.	68	53	35 (66%)	11	3 (27%)	1	–	3	1
2-4 yr.	90	41	22 (54%)	39	8 (20%)	9	4	1	1
>4 yr.	53*	28	18 (64%)	15	5 (33%)	9	2	–	–

*One patient with group unknown.

The Effect of Involvement of Lymph Nodes or Vein on Results. Another possible reason for the lack of decrease in recurrence rate in children receiving actinomycin-D could be that they had more extensive disease than those who did not receive it, although all patients were in Group I or II. Involvement of the renal vien or hilar nodes was more common in the patients who received actinomycin-D. Among eight such patients who received actinomycin-D, four developed distant metastases. In those children who did not receive actinomycin-D, two had node or vein involvement, and one got a distant metastasis. If patients who had involvement of the renal vein or lymph nodes are excluded from the two groups, there is still no difference in the incidence of recurrence of those who received actinomycin-D – nine of 29, and those who did not receive actinomycin-D – 11 of 33. Of the 11 patients with recurrences in the latter group, two developed a lesion in the other kidney (these were probably second primaries rather than metastases). If these two children are excluded, only nine of 33 developed metastases when no actinomycin-D was given.

It appears then that the groups are comparable and that the incidence of distant metastases is not affected by the administration of actinomycin-D to children in Group I or Group II.

Single vs Multiple Courses of Actinomycin-D. In 1967, Children's Cancer Group A compared the effect of a single course *vs* multiple courses of actinomycin-D on the incidence of metastases. To enter the study, the children had to be in Group I or II and also had to be over one year of age. One-half of the children were given a single course of actinomycin-D postoperatively and the other one-half, by card selection, received multiple courses of actinomycin-D starting immediately postoperatively, and then six and 12 weeks later, and then every three months for 18 months. The results of this study have recently been updated and are shown in the upper one-half of Table XII.

TABLE XII

Wilms' Tumor: Groups I and II Older Than One Year
Comparison of Influence of Actinomycin-D on Recurrence and Survival
CCGA Results Compared with Toronto Experience

	Actinomycin-D	Pts. Entered	Pts. Evaluated	Recurrences	Alive (after 4 yr.)
CCGA	Single Course	36	28	16 (57%)	20 (71%)
	Multiple Course	37	25	6 (24%)	20 (80%)
HSC + PMH	Single Course	29	29	11 (38%)	24 (83%)
	None (1920-68)	30	27*	13 (48%)	14 (52%)–(74%)**

*Three died of unrelated causes.
**Hypothetical – if pulmonary metastases had been treated.

Of those children who received a single course of actinomycin-D, 57% developed recurrences compared to 24% who were given multiple courses. On the basis of this study, the authors recommended that all children with Wilms' tumor be given multiple courses of actinomycin-D. Recently, however, it has become apparent that the percentage of patients alive four years after resection of the tumor is similar in both groups despite the difference in incidence of metastases. Those patients who developed metastases were treated in a variable manner at the discretion of the individual investigator, but usually with pulmonary radiation and actinomycin-D. Most of those who developed metastases have remained well so that the ultimate survival is similar for both groups of patients.

If, of our cases, we include only those who received a single course of actinomycin-D, who are over one year of age, and who are in Group I or II, we will then have a group of patients comparable to those of Children's Cancer Group A (CCGA). The incidence of distant or local recurrence in our cases is 38% and the four-year survival (83%) is similar to theirs (Table XII). This incidence of metastases, following a single course of actinomycin-D, is not significantly different from the incidence after multiple or single courses in the CCGA study. In fact, when our children in Group I and II who had no actinomycin-D are examined, the incidence of recurrences is not significantly different.

In order to collect enough children who fit the same criteria for age, operation and radiation as those in CCGA study *but* did not receive actinomycin-D, all eligible cases since 1920 were included. The incidence of recurrence in 27 such patients was 48%. The four-year survival in the 27 who were not given actinomycin-D is lower because, although the incidence of metastases was the same, no patient with metastases survived – a reflection of the inadequate treatment in the earlier years. At least 50% of children with pulmonary metastases can be expected to live at least four years after pulmonary radiation and actinomycin-D, and if 50% of those with metastases survive, the four-year survival would be 74% – equivalent to that in the Children's Cancer Group A Study.

DISCUSSION

The dramatic increase in survival in Wilms' tumor is due to multiple factors and not solely to actinomycin-D. Actinomycin-D does not appear to have influenced the incidence of distant or local recurrence in Groups I and II in our series. It is not possible to assess its value in Groups III and IV because a radical change in the radiotherapy took place shortly before the introduction of actinomycin-D and we cannot separate the effect of the improved radiation from that of the actinomycin-D.

The role of actinomycin-D in the treatment of pulmonary metastases is not clear. Too few children were treated with adequate pulmonary radiation alone to assess the effect of the addition of actinomycin-D. The Southwest Cancer Chemotherapy Group has reported similar good results in children with pulmonary metastases treated with pulmonary radiation and intravenous vincristine. If actinomycin-D does increase survival after pulmonary metastases develop, it appears that this effect is not unique but is shared by at least vincristine.

Current programs tend to add more chemotherapy to the treatment of Wilms' tumor. Multiple courses of actinomycin-D have almost become routine and recently vincristine is being given as well. Actinomycin-D is not without toxicity. Its immediate effects are vomiting, diarrhea, mouth ulcers and pancytopenia. It can cause liver toxicity and it increases skin reaction to radiation. It causes immunosuppression and the child is more susceptible to intercurrent disease. Its long-term effects on the chromosomes are not known.

If 60% of children are not going to develop metastases and if over one-half of those who get metastases can be salvaged, it is questionable whether we should subject children in Groups I or II to multiple courses of actinomycin-D without stronger proof that it is helpful. It is equally questionable whether even a single course is justified for children in Group I or II.

CONCLUSION

Improvements in surgery, radiotherapy, chemotherapy, and more careful follow-up of the patients, combined with an aggressive approach to the treatment of metastases, has improved the survival of children with Wilms' tumor, irrespective of the extent of the tumor at the time of diagnosis. Five years after diagnosis, 75% of children in Groups I and II, and 50% of children with residual disease in the abdomen are alive and well. Six of the 12 children who had distant metastases at the time of diagnosis are alive and free of disease four years later, and three of the four children with bilateral tumors at the time of diagnosis have survived five years.

In children with localized, resected tumors, controlled clinical trials are needed to evaluate the contribution of chemotherapy.

NEONATAL RENAL TUMORS

J. F. K. MANCER, M.D., B.Sc.(Med.), F.R.C.P.(C)*

The tumor registry at the Hospital for Sick Children (HSC) from 1924 to 1972 lists 43 renal tumors which presented when the patient was less than one year of age. Of the six tumors that presented in the neonatal period (when the patient was less than one month of age), five belonged to the entity known variously as fetal mesodermal hamartoma (FMH), congenital mesoblastic nephroma, or leiomyoma of the kidney. The five patients with FMH are all alive, free of tumor and have had follow-up studies made at periods ranging from 19 months to 13 years. The sixth neonatal tumor, a Wilms' tumor, was an incidental post mortem finding in a premature infant who died of hyaline membrane disease. The other 37 patients all had Wilms' tumor.

PATHOLOGICAL FINDINGS

Fetal Mesodermal Hamartoma

The detailed clinical and pathological data for the five cases of FMH are shown in Table I. The presenting symptom in four of the five patients was a palpable abdominal mass. The infant whose presenting symptom was hematuria, had an abdominal mass on physical examination.

All the tumors were 5 cm. or more in diameter and tended to be firm, rubbery and spherical. Each was large relative to the remainder of the kidney. The large size of the tumor left the uninvolved part of the kidney as a thin, stretched mass, splayed out on one side of the tumor. The cut surface resembled that of the common uterine leiomyoma, and had a whorled, bulging appearance and no definite encapsulation. The tumors varied from pale yellow-grey to white, with no evidence of hemorrhage or necrosis (Fig. 1).

The histological appearance varied, but mainly consisted of whorled bundles of smooth muscle cells (Figs. 2,3). One of the tumors had numerous mitotic figures and, although the cells were not completely mature, they were still identifiable as smooth muscle. The lesion was considered to be histologically benign. Mitoses were rare in the remaining tumors.

---

*Department of Pathology, The Hospital for Sick Children, Toronto.

TABLE I

Clinical and Pathological Data in Five Infants with FMH

Case number	1	2	3	4	5
Year of Diagnosis	1959	1960	1961	1970	1971
Age (days)	30	1	21	15	1
Sex	F	M	F	M	F
Presenting complaints:					
Abdominal mass	+	+	+	+	+
Hematuria	+	–	–	–	–
Tumor diameter (cm.)	5	6	7	5	5
Microscopic findings:					
Smooth muscle	+	+	+	+	+
Cartilage	–	+	–	+	–
Dysplasia	–	+	–	+	–
Hematopoiesis	–	+	+	–	–
Nephrectomy	+	+	+	+	+
Radiotherapy	Post-op	–	–	–	–
Recurrence	–	–	–	–	–
Follow-up (years)	13	12	10	2	1
Original diagnosis	Wilms'	Wilms'	Wilms'	FMH	FMH

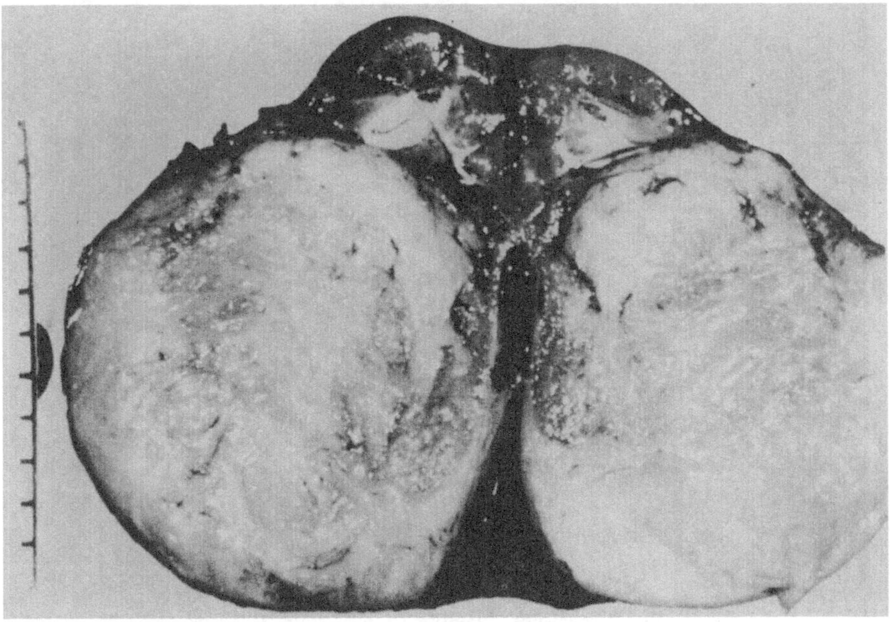

Fig. 1. Gross appearance of a typical fetal mesodermal hamartoma (Case 2).

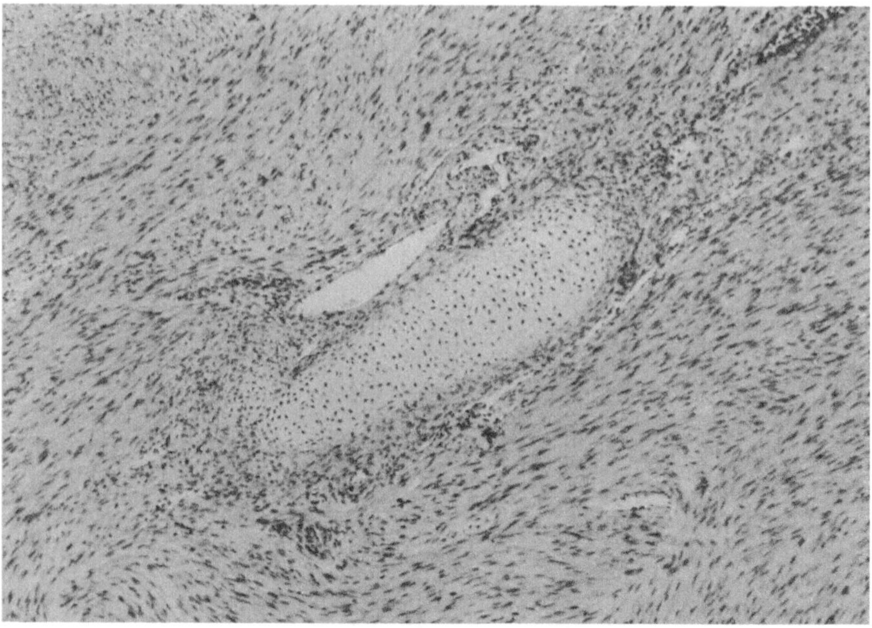

Fig. 2. Fetal mesodermal hamartoma (Case 2): interlacing bundles of smooth muscle cells with a central focus of hyaline cartilage (x115).

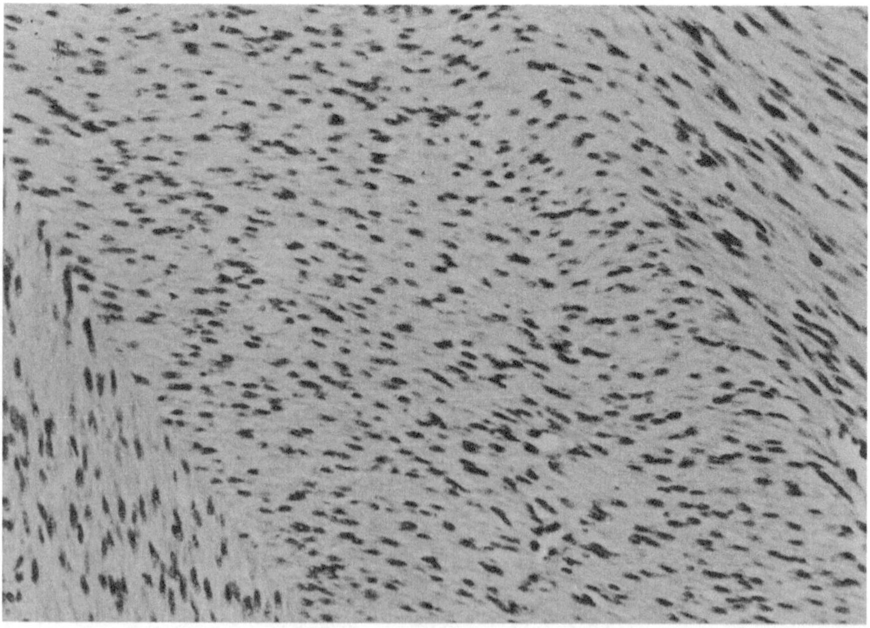

Fig. 3. Fetal mesodermal hamartoma: magnification of smooth muscle cells, illustrated in Fig. 2 (x290).

In all cases the edges of the tumor were poorly defined. Renal tubules were present within the lesions, but there was no evidence that the tubules had differentiated from the tumor. The tumor's smooth muscle cells tended to surround pre-existing renal tubules. Deeper, but still near the periphery of the tumor, there were larger masses of well-differentiated glomerular and tubular tissue, which had apparently been trapped by the proliferating lesion. In these areas, the glomeruli occasionally showed cystic dilation and had rudimentary glomerular tufts, giving the appearance of dysplastic renal tissue. Small foci of hyaline cartilage (Fig. 2) were present among the tumor cells, but only near regions of trapped renal tissue. The cartilage gradually merged into smooth muscle. The dysplastic changes in the engulfed renal tissue were probably due to distal obstruction of the dysplastic nephrons or the collecting system by the tumor. In all cases the tumor completely obscured the capsule and extended into the perirenal fat, surrounding fat cells at its periphery. If the tumor extended to the renal pelvis, the epithelium was unbroken by the tumor. Extramedullary hematopoesis was noted in two of the five cases.

All five patients were treated by nephrectomy. One patient also received postoperative radiotherapy, because the original histologic diagnosis was Wilms' tumor. Although the tumors in two other patients were originally diagnosed as Wilms' tumor, radiotherapy was not given because the tumor appeared well-differentiated in each case. In those cases where the original diagnosis was FMH, the patient did not receive radiotherapy. None of the patients was treated with chemotherapy.

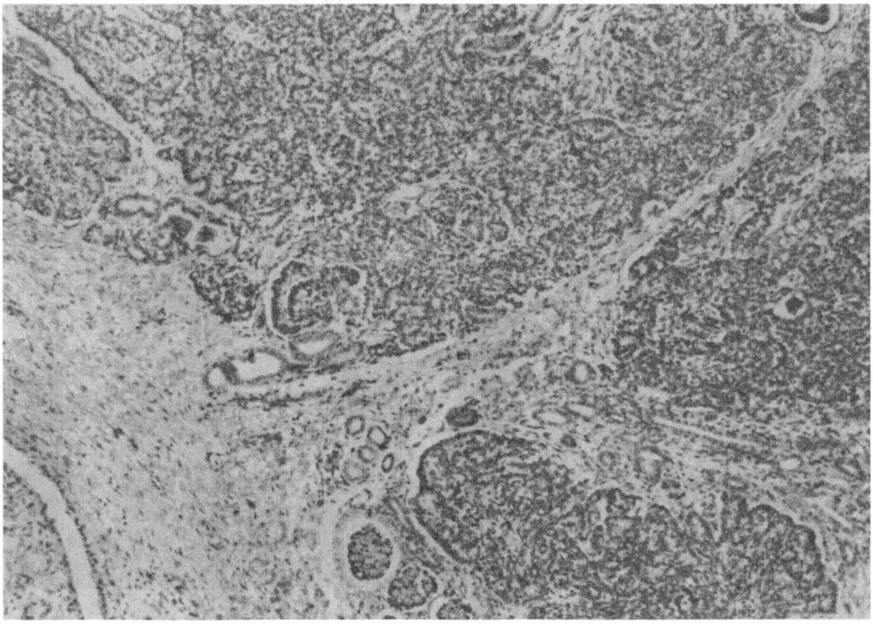

Fig. 4. Wilms' tumor, an incidental post mortem finding in a premature newborn who died of hyaline membrane disease (x115.)

Wilms' Tumor

In the single neonatal Wilms' tumor (Fig. 4), the tumor was well-differentiated and in an early stage of development. It was multifocal and bilateral, the largest focus being 8 mm. in diameter. The kidneys were only slightly enlarged although they were palpable clinically. There was no evidence of metastasis or vascular invasion. The tumor did not contribute to the patient's death, which was due to hyaline membrane disease. The patient was delivered by Cesarean section, because the mother had terminal carcinoma of the rectum.

DISCUSSION

FMH accounts for most of the renal tumors which present in the neonatal period but is infrequent in infants older than four weeks. Wilms' tumor is rare in infancy. Wigger[1], in his review of the literature, included a definite case of Wilms' tumor in an infant aged two months[2], and he considered it to be the youngest definite Wilms' tumor. This present series includes a neonatal Wilms' tumor but the patient did not present with signs and symptoms referable to the renal lesion. At HSC, the youngest child with Wilms' tumor that presented with renal signs or symptoms was three months of age.

In Bolande's series[3], six of 12 renal tumors presenting in patients under one year of age were FMH. In this series, Wilms' tumor had a higher incidence, 38 of 43 cases. Renal tumors in neonates are likely to be FMH and those in children over three months of age are likely to be Wilms' tumor. Renal tumors rarely occur in infants between one and three months of age (Figs. 5,6).

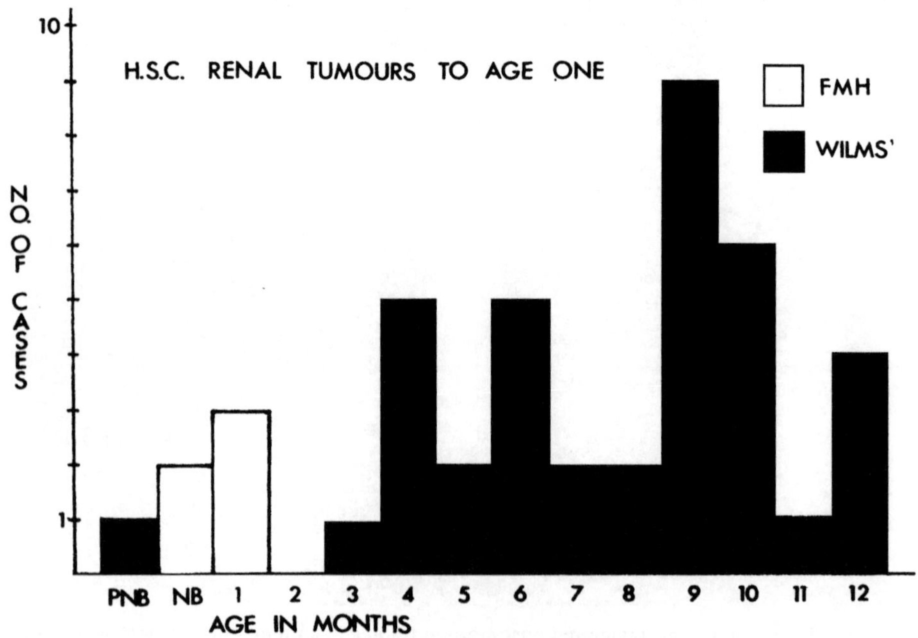

Fig. 5. Incidence of renal tumors in children one year of age and under, at the Hospital for Sick Children, Toronto.

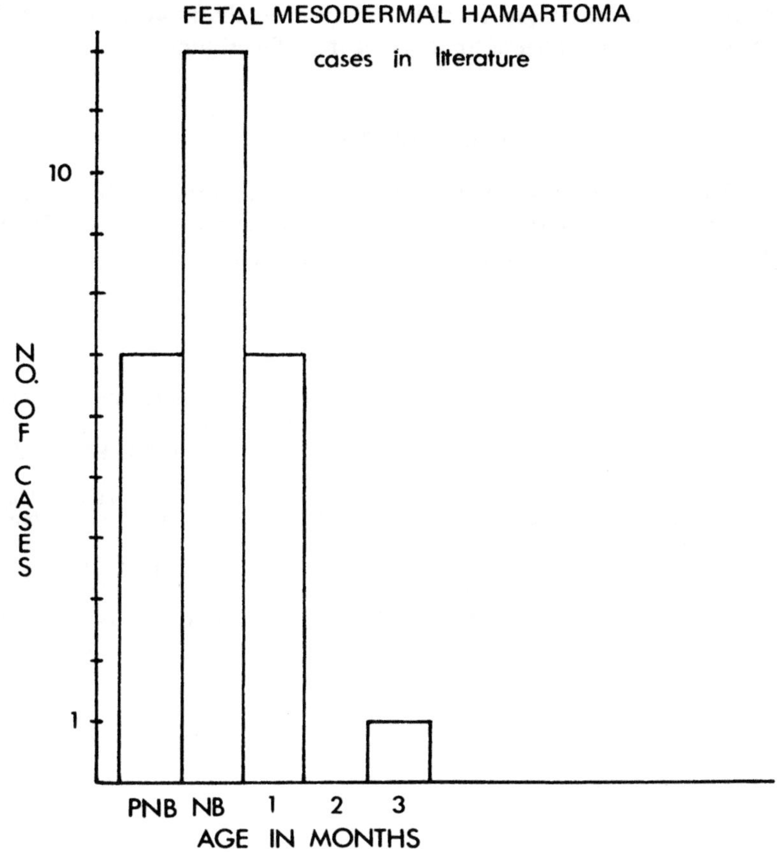

Fig. 6. Incidence of FMH in children, three months of age and under, from the literature.

Although FMH had been previously reported correctly as leiomyoma[4] and leiomyomatous hamartoma[5], Bolande *et al.* in 1967 emphasized that, in many cases, FMH had been misdiagnosed as Wilms' tumor. Wigger, in his review of FMH, discussed 22 pulished cases, eight of which were originally reported as Wilms' tumor and the remainder as sarcoma, leiomyoma, hamartoma or congenital mesoblastic nephroma. He added a further five cases of his own, three of which were originally diagnosed as Wilms' tumor.

The survival data in this and other series, and the absence of any reported cases with metastasis or recurrence following nephrectomy, indicate that FMH is a benign lesion. Although there were no postoperative deaths in this present series, Wigger's review includes reports of four deaths, two from surgical complications and one each attributed to chemotherapy and to sepsis associated with chemotherapy[1].

Nephrectomy alone, done under optimum conditions, is the most appropriate treatment. When the patient is a neonate and the surgical risk is considerable, the operation can be safely delayed on the assumption that the lesion is a fetal mesodermal hamartoma rather than Wilms' tumor.

CONCLUSIONS

Fetal mesodermal hamartoma is the most frequent renal tumor in the neonate.

It is important to differentiate between this benign tumor and Wilms' tumor, which rarely occurs before the third month of life.

REFERENCES

1 WIGGER, H. J.: Fetal hamartoma of the kidney: A benign, symptomatic, congenital tumor, not a form of Wilms' tumor. *Am J Clin Pathol,* **51:** 323, 1969.

2 LATTIMER, J. K., MELICOW, M. M. and USON, A. C.: Wilms' tumour: A report of 71 cases. *J Urol,* **80:** 401, 1958.

3 BOLANDE, R. P., BROUGH, A. J. and IZANT, R. J. Jr.: Congenital mesoblastic nephroma of infancy: A report of eight cases and the relationship to Wilms' tumor. *Pediatrics,* **40:** 272, 1967.

4 ZUCKERMAN, I. C., KERSHNER, D., LAYTNER, B. D. and HIRSCHL, D.: Leiomyoma of the kidney. *Ann Surg,* **126:** 220, 1947.

5 KAY, S., PRATT, C. B. and SALZBERG, A. M.: Hamartoma (leiomyatous type) of the kidney. *Cancer,* **19:** 1825, 1966.

THE NATIONAL WILMS' TUMOR STUDY: A PROGRESS REPORT*

GIULIO J. D'ANGIO, M.D., J. BRUCE BECKWITH, M.D., HARRY C. BISHOP, M.D., NORMAN BRESLOW, Ph.D., AUDREY E. EVANS, M.D., WILLARD E. GOODWIN, M.D., LOWELL R. KING, M.D., LAWRENCE K. PICKETT, M.D., LUCIUS F. SINKS, M.D., WATARU W. SUTOW, M.D. and JAMES A. WOLFF, M.D.**

Wilms' tumor was virtually incurable before pediatric surgeons, notably Ladd[1], perfected their surgical techniques. Steady improvements thereafter added radiation therapy[2] and chemotherapy. The routine postoperative use of actinomycin-D, as reported by Farber[3], produced a two-year survival rate of 81% in patients managed from the outset by an experienced team using combination therapy. Wolff and his colleagues[4] demonstrated the value of cyclic actinomycin-D given over a prolonged period after operation, and others[5,6] showed that vincristine sulfate was effective in the management of these children.

Surgery, radiation therapy and chemotherapy all have deleterious consequences, however. Irradiation particularly disrupts the growth and development of children[7]. Anti-mitotic chemical agents probably have similar untoward late effects. Therefore, pediatric oncologists have expressed concern about the routine use of several modes of therapy in all children with Wilms' tumor. Schneider in 1958, for example, questioned the need for postoperative radiation in children with well-localized and totally removed tumors[8]. Many sought to refine therapeutic programs, but no one centre – however large – can accumulate enough patients to study systematically the several points that required elucidation.

DESIGN OF THE NATIONAL STUDY

In 1969, investigators who were participating in national co-operative trials banded together to form the National Wilms' Tumor Study Group so that they could accumulate large numbers of patients and reach statistically meaningful results at the earliest possible moment. The founding organizations included Acute Leukemia Group B, Children's Cancer Study Group A, and Southwest Cancer Chemotherapy Study Group. Other institutions, not members of one of the organized study groups, also have joined the Study. The questions to be answered by the investigation were defined as follows:

---

*Supported in part by U.S.P.H.S. Grant No. R10 CA 11722.

**Appendix I shows the authors' affiliations.

1. Is postoperative radiation necessary for patients with well-encapsulated, localized lesions after what appears to be total removal?
2. Which of the two chemotherapeutic agents known to be effective against Wilms' tumor gives the better result; and can this result be improved by their combined use?

As secondary objectives, the Study sought to understand better the neoplasm and the neoplastic process through careful pathologic evaluation of the specimen both grossly and histologically; and by obtaining epidemiological data regarding possible associated diseases in the patients and in their families.

All patients are placed in specific groups according to the extent of their disease determined by individual clinical, roentgen and pathologic evaluation.

Group I: Tumor Limited to Kidney and Completely Resected. The surface of the renal capsule is intact. The tumor was not ruptured before or during removal. There is no residual tumor apparent beyond the margins of resection.

Group II: Tumor Extends Beyond the Kidney but is Completely Resected. There is local extension of the tumor, i.e., penetration beyond the pseudocapsule into the perirenal soft tissues, or periaortic lymph-node involvement. The renal vessels outside the kidney substance are infiltrated or contain tumor thrombus. There is no residual tumor apparent beyond the margins of resection.

Group III: Residual Non-Hematogenous Tumor Confined to Abdomen. Any one or more of the following:

1. The tumor has been biopsied or ruptured before or during operation.
2. There are implants on peritoneal surfaces.
3. Lymph nodes are involved beyond the abdominal periaortic chains.
4. The tumor is not completely resectable because of local infiltration into vital structures.

Group IV: Hematogenous Metastases. Deposits beyond Group III, e.g., lung, liver, bone and brain.

Group V: Bilateral Renal Involvement Either Initially or Subsequently.

It should be noted that the schema given above employs various criteria that were thought to have prognostic significance so that patients could be categorized and treated accordingly. However, these criteria have not yet been shown to have prognostic significance, so that the word "group" rather than "stage" has been adopted. It should also be noted that Group V patients are not randomized because the numbers are too small and, furthermore, these children present especially difficult clinical problems which require individual attention.

The organization of the Study is shown in Fig. 1. A detailed exposition of the protocol has been published elsewhere[9].

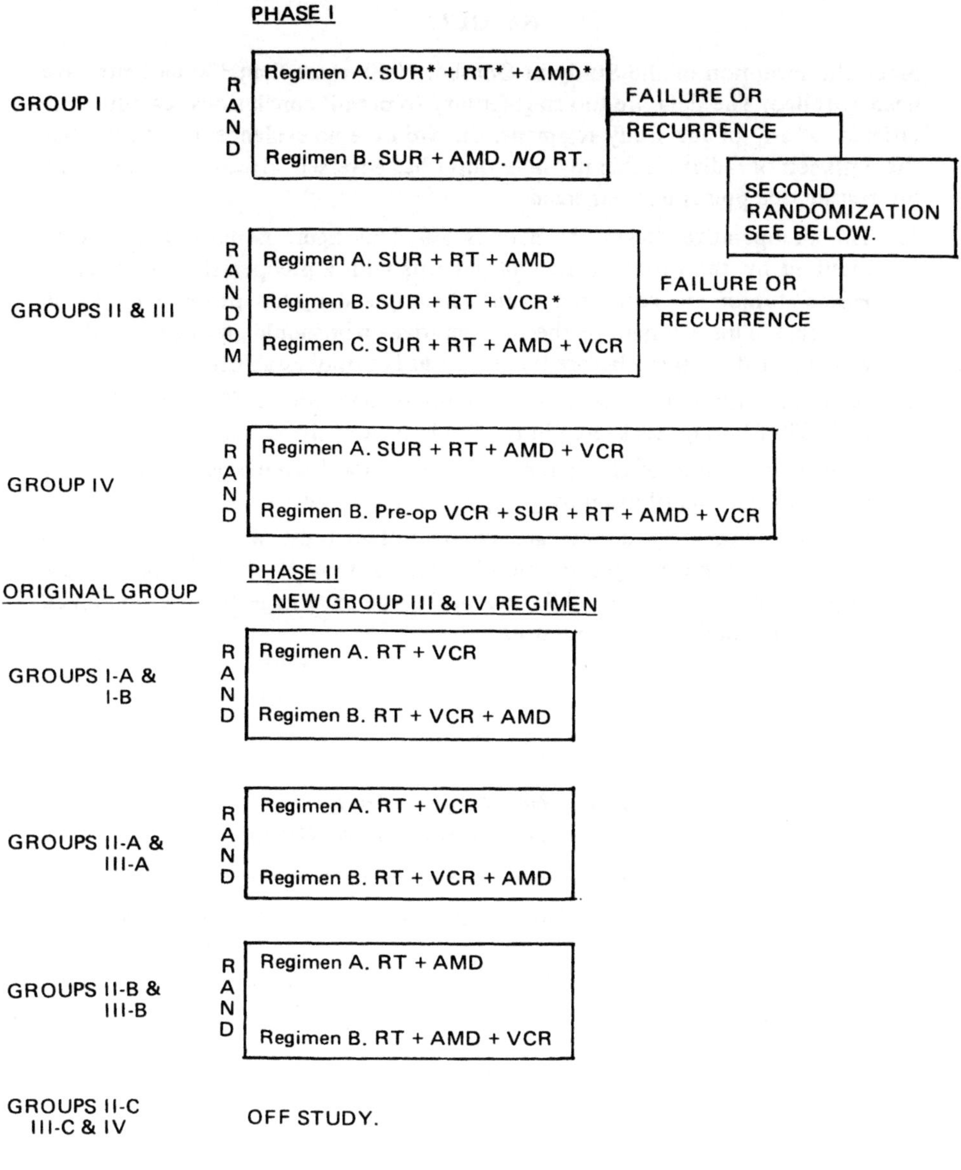

*SUR = Surgery RT = Radiotherapy AMD = Actinomycin-D VCR = Vincristine

Fig. 1. Organization of the Wilms' Tumor Study.

RESULTS

Since the inception of the Study in October 1969, more than 300 patients have been enrolled. The data are too fragmentary to permit conclusions regarding the efficacy of any of the study regimens, but we have no evidence to indicate that the omission of radiation therapy in Group I has adversely affected results. Some interesting side points have emerged:

1. The preoperative diagnostic error is 6%. This figure is derived from data required by the protocol, i.e., all patients with a preoperative diagnosis of Wilms' tumor are registered even when this diagnosis proves later to be incorrect. This estimate of the preoperative error should give pause to those who advocate therapy before the diagnosis is firmly established.
2. Bilateral tumors are relatively uncommon; only about 5% of all children with Wilms' tumor registered in the Study have such lesions.
3. A high proportion of children have relatively localized disease at the time of diagnosis. The distribution by group is shown in Table I.
4. Children with early disease are younger than those with more advanced tumors. The mean ages in months for Groups I, II, III, and IV are respectively 30.5, 39.9, 37.9, and 66.1. The mean age for the combined patient population is 40.0 months.

TABLE I

National Wilms' Tumor Study: Distribution of Children Among Five Groups

Group	No. of Patients Entered	% of Patients Entered
I	83	42
II	48	25
III	39	20
IV	17	9
I/II, III*	8	4
Total	195	

*This designation indicates patients believed by the surgeon at operation to have well-localized tumors and grossly to qualify as Group I but found on histologic examination of the specimen to have more advanced, albeit still localized, disease.

All those interested in the management of children with cancer are indebted to the many investigators in several different specialties who have combined their efforts in this Study. The contribution they are making to our understanding of the disease and its optimum treatment will benefit many children in the years to come.

ACKNOWLEDGEMENTS

The Study is made possible by the co-operation and dedication of the many investigators enrolled in Acute Leukemia Group B; Children's Cancer Study Group A; Southwest Cancer Chemotherapy Study Group; and Southern California Kaiser-Permanente, Los Angeles; Stanford University School of Medicine, Palo Alto; Presbyterian-St. Luke's Hospital, Chicago; Johns Hopkins Hospital, Baltimore; Tulane-Charity Hospital, New Orleans; Touro Infirmary, New Orleans; Albany Medical Center Hospital, Albany; Izaak Walton Killam Hospital, Halifax, Nova Scotia; St. Christopher's Hospital, Philadelphia; Saskatoon Cancer Clinic, Saskatchewan; Medical University of South Carolina; and Children's Hospital of Michigan, Detroit. This study would not be possible without the contributions they make, and the co-ordinating and administrative assistance supplied by the American Academy of Pediatrics which sponsors the Study.

REFERENCES

1 LADD, W. E.: Embryoma of the kidney (Wilms' tumor). *Ann Surg,* **108**:885, 1938.

2 GROSS, R. E. and NEUHAUSER, E. B. D.: Treatment of mixed tumors of the kidneys in childhood. *Pediatrics,* **6**: 843, 1950.

3 FARBER, S.: Chemotherapy in the treatment of leukemia and Wilms' tumor. *JAMA,* **198**:826, 1966.

4 WOLFF, J. A., KRIVIT, W., NEWTON, W. A., Jr. and D'ANGIO, G. J.: Single *vs.* multiple dose dactinomycin therapy of Wilms' tumor. A controlled co-operative study conducted by the Children's Cancer Study Group A. *N Engl J Med,* **279**:290, 1968.

5 SULLIVAN, M. P., SUTOW, W. W., CANGIR, A. and TAYLOR, G.: Vincristine sulfate in management of Wilms' tumor. *JAMA,* **202**:381, 1967.

6 VIETTI, T. J., SULLIVAN, M. P., HAGGARD, M. E., HOLCOMB, T. M. and BERRY, D. H.: Vincristine sulfate and radiation therapy in metastatic Wilms' tumor. *Cancer,* **25**:12, 1970.

7 VAETH, J. M., ed.: Frontiers of Radiation Therapy and Oncology – Radiation Effect and Tolerance. Normal Tissue. Vol. 6, S. Karger, Basel, Switzerland, 1972.

8 SCHNEIDER, M.: Renal embryoma. *In:* Progress in Radiation Therapy, edited by F. Buschke, Grune & Stratton, New York, 1958, p.180.

9 D'ANGIO, G. J., BECKWITH, J. B., BISHOP, H. C., BRESLOW, N., EVANS, A. E., GOODWIN, W., KING, L. R., PICKETT, L. K., SINKS, L., SUTOW, W. W. and WOLFF, J. A.: The National Wilms' Tumor Study: A Progress Report. *Cancer.* (In press)

APPENDIX I

National Wilms' Tumor Study Committee Members

Name	Institution	Specialty	Parent Group Represented & Term†
Beckwith, J. Bruce	Children's Orthopedic Hospital, Seattle	Pathology	Pediatric Pathologists Club
Bishop, Harry C.	Children's Hospital of Philadelphia	Pediatric Surgery	Surgical Section, Amer. Acad. of Ped. (AAP)
Breslow, Norman	University of Washington Seattle	Biostatistics	
*D'Angio, Giulio J.	Memorial Hospital, New York	Radiology	Soc. Ped. Rad., Am. Soc. Ther. Rad.
**Evans, Audrey E.	Children's Hospital of Philadelphia	Pediatrics	Independent Group
Goodwin, Willard E.	University of California at Los Angeles	Urology	Urology Section of the AAP
King, Lowell R.	St. Luke's-Presbyterian Hospital, Chicago	Urology	Urology Section of the AAP
Pickett, Lawrence K.	Yale University School of Medicine, New Haven	Pediatric Surgery	Surgical Section of the AAP
Sinks, Lucius F.	Roswell Park Memorial Institute, Buffalo	Pediatrics	Acute Leukemia Group B
Sutow, Wataru W.	M. D. Anderson Hospital, Houston	Pediatrics	Southwest Cancer Chemotherapy Study Group
Wolff, James A.	Babies Hospital, New York	Pediatrics	Children's Cancer Study Group A

Statistical Centre: Department of Biostatistics, RD 92, University of Washington, Seattle, Washington 98105

Randomization Centre: The Children's Hospital of Philadelphia, 1740 Bainbridge St., Philadelphia, Pa. 19146

*Chairman.

**Co-ordinator.

†All Committee members term of office has been 1969 to the present except for Dr. L. R. King (1969-1971) and Dr. W. E. Goodwin (1971-present).

PANEL ON WILMS' TUMOR

Moderator: J. M. M. DARTE*
Panelists: G. J. D'ANGIO**, R. D. JEFFS†,
R. D. T. JENKIN‡, and M. J. SONLEY‡

Question: In view of the data that has just been presented, how do you now treat Wilms' tumor?

Dr. Sonley: We have not been able to demonstrate by retrospective studies that actinomycin-D has improved survival in localized resectable Wilms' tumor. In this situation we do not use maintenance therapy but, whenever irradiation is employed, give a single intravenous course of actinomycin-D – 15 μg./kg. on each of the first five days of irradiation.

When there has been tumor spill at operation, or there is residual or metastatic disease, or in any child in whom the outlook seems bad, we irradiate the whole abdomen postoperatively, and add an initial course of actinomycin-D and six weekly injections of vincristine. Maintenance actinomycin-D and vincristine is given every three months for 18 months.

We are looking at these programs critically to see whether we can reduce the amount of elective chemotherapy now employed.

Dr. Jenkin: The value of actinomycin-D is most clearly seen in the management of the child who relapses with pulmonary metastases alone. Total-lung irradiation alone (2000 rads/28 days: 270 Kv) offers only a 15% cure rate, while the same irradiation combined with a five-day course of actinomycin-D gives a cure rate better than 50%. It may be that maintained combination therapy will push the cure rate higher. It seems that this increased ability to salvage children with pulmonary metastases is the main factor in the current improvement in cure rates.

Dr. Sonley: The improved results in lung metastases with irradiation and actinomycin-D do not necessarily provide evidence of mutual potentiation. Equally good results have been obtained by the Southwestern Chemotherapy Group with irradiation and vincristine: nine of 14 children alive three years after development of pulmonary metastases.

*Charles A. Janeway Child Health Centre, St. John's, Newfoundland.
**Memorial Hospital for Cancer and Allied Diseases, New York, N.Y., U.S.A.
†The Hospital for Sick Children, Toronto.
‡The Princess Margaret Hospital, Toronto.
‡The Princess Margaret Hospital, Toronto.

Dr. Darte: What about Group I patients?

Dr. Sonley: At present we use local tumor-bed irradiation postoperatively combined with actinomycin-D. However, we should look at this program to see if we can decrease this combined treatment further or omit it altogether in some patients.

Dr. Jenkin: It is important not to overtreat a child with Wilms' tumor. More than 60% of these children can be cured by operation, irradiation and unmaintained actinomycin-D. If we institute maintained combination chemotherapy regimens in all these patients, we will treat 60% unnecessarily.

The late effects of these combined programs are unknown, but as you have heard today, children do die as a result of treatment for Wilms' tumor. I believe that only high-risk patients should be subjected to such protocols.

Question: Why do you irradiate the whole abdomen in so many of your patients?

Dr. Jenkin: At present we irradiate the whole abdomen in children with Group III or IV tumors, and boys in Group II. In girls, in Group II, we omit the pelvis in order to avoid irradiating the ovaries.

Since Wilms' tumor tends to be confined to the abdomen, or, at a later date, to the thorax, we prefer to irradiate the whole compartment. There is no good evidence that results in Wilms' tumor are dose-dependent above a medium dose range, e.g., 2500 rads/28 days. At this level, it is practical to irradiate the whole abdomen, with appropriate shielding of the remaining kidney, without appreciable morbidity.

I suspect that, in several childhood tumors, the volume irradiated is more critical than the dose, and that tumor recurrence may often be due to an inadequate treatment volume rather than to an inadequate dose. Having offered this opinion, I admit there are no hard data in Wilms' tumor to indicate either the optimal volume or dose, and that equally good results have been obtained with other treatment regimens. Certainly abdominal recurrence is uncommon when large-field, moderate-dose methods are employed.

In a childhood tumor with a high cure rate, the late effects of the irradiation will be demonstrated inexorably and in full. For this reason and because we have achieved results as good as any, we prefer to give moderate doses until we have good evidence to the contrary.

Dr. D'Angio: May I comment? Since this is such a modest dose, maybe it is not contributing to survival at all, and perhaps the best dose is zero? With present-day surgery, abdominal recurrence in Groups I and II would be uncommon even without postoperative irradiation. Since relapse in the lung is the main problem, systemic therapy is more appealing intellectually than local therapy. The Group I tumors, once we are satisfied that we can accurately define a truly localized tumor, may require operation as the only treatment. I believe this group should be studied in a prospective randomized trial to determine the value of elective actinomycin-D.

A Group A study, which compared single and maintained courses of actinomycin-D, remains the only prospective, randomized trial and, as such, must be given due weight when compared with retrospective experience.

Let me emphasize that our whole effort in the National Wilms' Tumor Study (NWTS) is to refine methods of therapy. We may well establish that, in Group I, local postoperative irradiation is unnecessary when actinomycin-D is given. The next generation study would be to determine whether or not chemotherapy is needed in Group I. At present, patients, who fail in Group I, fail because of pulmonary metastases.

Finally, the Group A study demonstrated that, while survival with maintenance actinomycin-D was not statistically better than a single course, recurrence rate was lower with maintenance therapy. Sometimes you have to work very hard to salvage the child who relapses and at a high cost in morbidity whether due to the operation, irradiation or chemotherapy. Is it better to overtreat a proportion of these children to spare those that will require the sometimes horrendous attack necessary to bring them back?

We are all trying to devise systems of therapy that are good for every man to apply. At present the child with a Wilms' tumor should be sent to a cancer centre so that methods, which will be applicable in any institution, can be evolved. What we are after in the long run are treatment methods that can be applied in the local community.

Dr. Jeffs: In the National Wilms' Tumor Study why is there not a third category in Group I – surgery alone?

Dr. D'Angio: Practical considerations. It would take too long to accumulate the patients.

Dr. Jeffs: And the duration of a two-arm study?

Dr. D'Angio: It is projected at 20 years. I think it will be less.

Dr. Jeffs: What late effects of irradiation have been seen in Toronto?

Dr. Jenkin: In frequency and degree, the late effects are dose dependent. The moderate dose – large volume method we employ produces some decrease in growth in the irradiated volume. The sitting height is reduced a little, but this is not clinically apparent and must be sought to be detected. Patients treated since 1958 have had minimal scoliosis and it has not become a clinical problem.

Certainly this treatment involves a risk of late induced malignancy but the exact degree of that risk is unknown. We have not yet induced a malignancy in any child in the series just described, but we must expect a slightly higher incidence of the common abdominal malignancies when the child reaches middle and old age.

Dr. Sonley: We do see osteochondromas in the irradiated area occasionally, particularly at the costochondral junctions, the iliac crest and the scapula. So far, these have been only cosmetic problems.

Dr. Jenkin: We are concerned about the late effects of irradiation on the remaining kidney because, during whole abdominal irradiation, it receives approximately 1250 rads over 28 days. We really do not know what long-term effects 1250 rads will have on the kidney. While we have had no serious long-term effects to date, it is possible that these children may risk chronic nephritis some decades later.

Dr. Schweisguth: What problems have you had with subsequent ovarian function?

Dr. Jenkin: When the ovaries receive 2500 rads over 28 days, it must induce major functional impairment but, despite this, we have had patients pass through menarche and subsequently menstruate normally. More often menarche will be delayed or there will be primary amenorrhea. We have not followed enough girls with advanced disease for long enough periods to determine the relative probabilities. We have no evidence about fertility though we assume this treatment causes infertility.

Dr. Wilbur: What late effects may be expected from actinomycin-D or vincristine?

Dr. D'Angio: This is a very important question. We have just been granted a contract by the National Cancer Institute in Washington to investigate the late effects following irradiation and/or chemotherapy in Wilms' tumor and choriocarcinoma. Late effects on organ function; psychosocial factors; oncogenesis – these areas are all important.

Dr. Tefft, in reviewing the Boston Children's Hospital experience, found that 2% of previously irradiated children developed second tumors. Therefore, children who have been irradiated should have a lifetime follow-up if they are to be adequately screened for late effects.

Dr. Jeffs: We have been concentrating on medical management. The problem of preoperative assessment and of making a correct diagnosis will always be with us.

A major improvement in survival rate at the Hospital for Sick Children occurred in about 1946 when we began to approach the renal vessels by way of a transverse abdominal incision. The survival rate rose from 17% to 45%, which has been improved further by the other modalities of treatment.

The question of whether to operate on an emergency basis has always interested us. Our more leisurely approach, investigation and operation within 48 hours of admission, does not appear to have adversely affected our results. Perhaps Dr. Gross' teaching, immediate surgery even in the middle of the night, may have to be modified.

Dr. D'Angio: As one of Dr. Gross' former internes, I should point out that by dramatizing immediate surgery, he drew attention to the deplorable situation that existed in those days when children might be on the ward for two to three weeks while people considered what to do. The point is that one should get on with the job and not waste time with unnecessary investigations.

Question: When do you begin postoperative irradiation?

Dr. Jenkin: Usually on the third, fourth or fifth postoperative day – as soon as the child is reasonably fit. There is no good evidence to favor irradiation on the day of surgery. I believe you do more harm than good if you start too soon.

Question: When do metastases appear?

Dr. Sonley: The median time was about five months and did not seem to depend on whether actinomycin-D had been given.

Dr. Darte: One last question?

Dr. Wilbur: What is the value of preoperative irradiation or preoperative vincristine?

Dr. Schweisguth: This question has yet to be answered. The International Society of Pediatric Oncology has organized a prospective randomized trial in Europe in which preoperative and postoperative irradiation are being compared. This should eventually answer your question. In my opinion, preoperative irradiation is a good way to start the treatment of large tumors and this seems to have been confirmed by our experience with 248 children treated at Villejuif.

Dr. D'Angio: How many false diagnoses of Wilms' tumor have you discovered in patients who received preoperative irradiation?

Dr. Schweisguth: About 8%. The most difficult differential diagnosis is that which involves the multicystic kidney.

Dr. D'Angio: In the National Wilms' Tumor Study, neuroblastoma was the commonest wrong diagnosis, so that in these children preoperative irradiation would not be unreasonable. However, having said that, I am against it!

Dr. Darte: I must stop discussion at this point though the panelists obviously have much more to contribute.

PATHOLOGY OF TUMORS OF THE TESTIS IN CHILDREN

DESMOND MAGNER, M.D., F.R.C.P.(C)*

According to Young *et al.*[1] 2 to 5% of testicular tumors occur in children. Collins and Pugh[2] found that, of 952 testicular tumors, 20 (2%) occurred in patients under 15 years of age and, of 22 paratesticular sarcomas, six (27%) were in children in this age group. At the Canadian Tumor Reference Centre, 31 (7%) of 456 testicular tumors and seven (29%) of 24 paratesticular sarcomas were in patients under 15 years. Table I shows the Reference Centre's series of 38 testicular and paratesticular tumors in children, grouped according to histologic type. Thirty-one were testicular neoplasms. Five of the six rhabdomyosarcomas and two of the three neoplasms listed as "other" were paratesticular.

TABLE I

Neoplasms of Testis and Paratesticular Tissues In Children

Histological Type	No. of Cases
Infantile adenocarcinoma	24
Rhabdomyosarcoma	6
Teratoma	3
Reticulum cell sarcoma	2
Other	3
Total	38

*Professor and Head, Department of Pathology, University of Ottawa; Director of Laboratories. Ottawa General Hospital; Registrar, Canadian Tumor Reference Centre, National Cancer Institute of Canada, Department of Pathology, University of Ottawa, Ottawa.

Bryant and I[3] reported briefly two of these tumors in 1951. In 1956 and 1962, in papers based on five and 13 patients, respectively, Campbell, Wiglesworth and I[4,5] asserted that the tumor was histologically distinctive and characteristic of infancy, and that prompt orchiectomy was often curative. White[6] in 1910 had given a clear account of this tumor under the name "carcinoma myxomatodes", but it had not been recognized as an entity before our 1956 paper. A few cases, however, had been reported usually under the name "embryonal carcinoma". In 1963, Abell and Holtz[7] challenged our view that the tumor was histologically distinctive and classified it as embryonal carcinoma, that is, as undifferentiated teratoma. They agreed, however that its behavior differed from that of embryonal carcinoma of adults, the prognosis being less grave. All who have written on this subject agree that the tumor usually occurs in boys, but Pierce *et al.*[8] in 1970 described it in an old man. Its histogenesis is uncertain and it may be either germinal or non-germinal. Consequently the tumor is known by a number of names, including infantile adenocarcinoma with clear cells[4,5], orchioblastoma[9], embryonal carcinoma[7], embryonal adenocarcinoma[1], endodermal sinus tumor[10] and yolk sac tumor[8]. Table II presents a brief review of the medical literature concerning this tumor.

On gross examination, the tumor expands the testis to a greater or lesser degree without breaching the tunica albuginea. It is pale yellowish-tan, solid or microcystic, with cut surfaces often covered with a layer of sticky fluid. Microscopically, the most characteristic feature is the presence of heavily vacuolated tumor cells arranged in loosely woven masses, irregular tubular spaces and forming small cystic cavities. Vacuoles often contain glycogen and sudanophilic material, and sometimes contain mucin, usually in small quantities.

Of the 24 cases we have studied, the age range at clinical onset was from four to 30 months, the median age being 17 months. Seventeen patients are alive and well one to 28 years after orchiectomy, 14 having survived for over four years. Seven are dead, survival after orchiectomy varying from two to 14 months. Of the 17 healthy patients, four had postoperative irradiation. Irradiation was given after orchiectomy in four of the seven infants who died but in two it was for palliation. The histological appearance of the tumors did not allow one to predict which patients would do well and which die. It may be worth noting that the median age at clinical onset was 14 months among the 17 survivors, and 22 months among the fatal cases. Pierce *et al.*[8] and Houser *et al.*[11] noted an increased mortality in patients two years of age or older, compared to those less than two years.

An autopsy was done in only one of our seven fatal cases. This child had no local recurrence and the pelvic tissues were free of tumor. Retroperitoneally there was a large mass of metastatic tumor which surrounded and depressed the left kidney and invaded the left psoas muscle and diaphragm. Tumor had invaded the left renal vein and extended into the inferior vena cava. A tumor embolus occluded the right pulmonary artery. The liver contained metastatic nodules. Young *et al.*[1] found no retroperitoneal lymph-node metastases in three

TABLE II

Infantile Adenocarcinoma of Testis – Historical Outline

Author and Year	Name of Tumor	Characteristic of Infancy	Distinctive Pattern	Distinctive Behaviour	Histogenesis
WHITE 1910	carcinoma myxomatodes	–	–	–	intratesticular ducts
MAGNER *et al.* 1951/56/63	adenocarcinoma with clear cells	yes	yes	yes	uncertain
TEOH *et al.* 1960	orchioblastoma	yes	yes	yes	testicular tubules
ABELL and HOLTZ 1963	embryonal carcinoma	no	no	yes	germinal cell
HUNTINGTON *et al.* 1963	endodermal sinus tumor (teilum)	predilection	yes	yes	extraembryonic mesoblast
YOUNG *et al.* 1970	embryonal adenocarcinoma	predilection	yes	yes	germinal cell

cases and suggested that this tumor may have a propensity for hematogenous spread, with lymphatic involvement occurring predominantly in advanced cases.

RHABDOMYOSARCOMA OF TESTIS AND PARATESTICULAR TISSUES

In four of our six cases, a localized mass arose, apparently from the tunica vaginalis, and compressed the testis. One tumor encased and compressed the testis and one was apparently intratesticular. Because the testis does not contain striated muscle one must consider whether this tumor could be a teratoma with a dominant striated muscle component. In one intratesticular rhabdomyosarcoma of childhood he reported, Davis[12], also considered this possibility. In four of our six cases cross striations were clearly visible in tumor cells; in the other two, this differentiation could not be made with light microscopy but otherwise the histology was entirely consistent with that of rhabdomyosarcoma.

The age range in our six cases was two to eight years. Only one child is known to have died from his tumor. The others survived without evidence of metastases for one to nine years (Table III).

TABLE III

Rhabdomyosarcoma of Childhood
Testicular and Paratesticular – 6 Cases
Treatment: Orchiectomy

Age (yr)	Site	Postop Course
3	Paratesticular	No recurrence – 1 yr
2	Paratesticular	No recurrence – 9 yr
6	Paratesticular	No recurrence – 5 yr
6	Paratesticular	Died – 1 yr
2	Paratesticular	No recurrence – 2 yr
8	Testicular	No recurrence – 5 yr

Holtz and Abell[13] described four childhood paratesticular rhabdomyosarcomas. Of these four children, three were healthy two, three and 12 years later; the fourth was alive with extensive metastases four months after operation. Treatment was orchiectomy in our six cases and in the four of Holtz and Abell[13]. Thus, of 10 childhood rhabdomyosarcomas with follow-up (one intratesticular and nine paratesticular), eight were alive and apparently well from one to 12 years after orchiectomy, one was alive but with metastases four months after operation, and one had died of his tumor.

TERATOMA OF TESTIS

Of 33 testicular and paratesticular neoplasms in infants and children described by Abell and Holtz[7], 10 were teratomas, two primary tumors being found in one patient (bilateral). Five tumors were of the adult type, five were partially differentiated. According to Houser *et al.*[11], teratomas account for one-quarter of germinal testicular tumors in infancy and childhood, the remainder consisting of the tumors we have called "infantile adenocarcinoma". In the Canadian Tumor Reference Centre, we have only three teratomas (Table IV).

TABLE IV

Teratoma of Testis in Childhood – 3 Cases
Treatment: Orchiectomy

Age (yr)	Histological Type	Postop Course
2	Adult	No recurrence – 7 yr
5	Partially differentiated	No recurrence – 3 yr
1/2	Adult	No recurrence – 1 yr

The three patients with this tumor in our series are all alive and well. The two adult tumors were cystic and composed of mature tissue from all germ layers. The partially differentiated tumor was solid and composed partly of adult tissue but largely of relatively undifferentiated epithelial and mesenchymal elements. Unlike teratomas in adults, in which even differentiated lesions may be fatal, teratomas in children, whether differentiated or not, seem to have a benign prognosis. None of the 27 patients with follow-up collected by Houser *et al.*[11], including the 10 reported by Abell and Holtz[7], is known to have died of his tumor. Eighteen patients have survived for from four to 30 years.

MALIGNANT LYMPHOMA OF TESTIS

Gowing[14] set forth the problem of primary lymphomas of the testis succinctly when he wrote "The question here is the same as that posed by lymphomas presenting as local tumor masses in other organs and tissues, namely, whether the tumor is truly primary at the site of presentation or whether it represents a precocious local development of an already disseminated disease". At the Canadian Tumor Reference Centre, we have collected 20 malignant lymphomas of the testis, which presented as primary testicular tumors. Two of these are in children (Table V) both nine years of age.

TABLE V

Malignant Lymphoma of Testis in Childhood – 2 Cases
Histological Type: Reticulum Cell

Age (Yr)	Treatment	Postop Course
9	Orchiectomy	No recurrence – 5 yr
9	Orchiectomy	No recurrence – 5 yr

Collins and Pugh[2] encountered 66 malignant testicular lymphomas, one of which occurred in a child under four years of age. In surveying the pertinent medical literature, it is not always easy to determine whether the lesions described presented as primary testicular neoplasms. However, Melicow[15] recorded a primary lymphosarcoma "or possibly localized lymphoid hyperplasia" in a seven-year-old boy; eight years after orchiectomy, he was healthy without evidence of recurrence or metastases. Waddell[16] described a lymphosarcoma in an eight-year-old who died shortly after operation, with clinical evidence of abdominal and pulmonary involvement. Turley and Moore[17] encountered a malignant lymphoma in an eight-year-old who died with an abdominal mass and pulmonary involvement four months after operation. Miller and Sharp[18] recorded a reticulum-cell sarcoma in a child of eight, who had no follow-up.

Our two patients with this lesion are alive without evidence of recurrence or metastases five years after operation. Neither received any treatment other than orchiectomy. The question is, are these tumors really malignant lymphomas or could they represent chronic granulomatous orchitis secondary to trauma, infection or autoimmune response. Microscopically, the lesions in our cases lacked the features of granulomatous orchitis namely, pleomorphic cellular infiltrate, diffuse increase in fibrous tissue and peritubular fibrosis. Furthermore, according to Gowing[14], granulomatous orchitis is a disease of the second one-half of life. If our cases are truly malignant lymphomas, Stout's[19] comment seems appropriate. He wrote "For me, lymphosarcoma seems to exhibit two different disease patterns . . . There is the more common lymphosarcoma that causes death in two, three or more years with multiple involvement and the altogether different variety that has the solitary or focal involvement and is not always followed by involvement of other areas. I do not know of any way to distinguish histologically between the two".

OTHER TUMORS OF THE TESTIS AND PARATESTICULAR TISSUES

Our series included one gonadal stromal tumor of Sertoli-cell type, one undifferentiated paratesticular sarcoma and one fibroma of the spermatic cord. All patients are now alive and well following orchiectomy, the patient with sarcoma having survived for six years.

COMMENT

Our series, like most other reported series of childhood testicular tumors, contained no seminomas. However, Thackray[20] described three seminomas in boys aged 12, 13 and 15 years. Interstitial-cell tumors are much more common. Houser *et al.*[11] collected 40 from the medical literature up to 1965. Our series contained none of these tumors and only one gonadal stromal tumor (Houser *et al.* [11] had collected 21). We may have had a disproportionately large number of infantile adenocarcinomas because many were sent to us by other pathologists so that we could confirm that the tumor was the type we had described.

Of our 38 tumors, 31 – 24 infantile adenocarcinomas, six rhabdomyosarcomas and one undifferentiated sarcoma – had undoubted malignant potential. It is noteworthy that treatment with orchiectomy was apparently curative in 24 of these young patients. The three teratomatous tumors behaved benignly as they are known to do in infancy. In view of the long survival of the two patients with tumors diagnosed as malignant lymphoma, the possibility cannot be excluded that these lesions are actually benign. On the other hand, these cases may represent localized malignant lymphomas cured by orchiectomy.

REFERENCES

1 YOUNG, P. G., MOUNT, B. M., FOOTE, F. W., Jr. and WHITMORE, F. W., Jr.: Embryonal adenocarcinoma in the prepubertal testis. A clinicopathologic study of 18 cases. *Cancer,* **26:** 1065, 1970.

2 COLLINS, D. H. and PUGH, R. C. B.: Classification and frequency of testicular tumours. *In:* The Pathology of Testicular Tumours. Studies from the Testicular Tumour Panel and Registry of the Pathological Society of Great Britain and Ireland in association with the British Empire Cancer Campaign for Research, edited by D. H. Collins and R. C. B. Pugh, E. & S. Livingstone Ltd., Edinburgh and London, 1965, p.1.

3 MAGNER, D. and BRYANT, A. J. S.: Adenocarcinoma of the testis occurring in infants. Report of two cases. *Arch Pathol,* **51:** 82, 1951.

4 MAGNER, D., CAMPBELL, J. S. and WIGLESWORTH, F. W.: Testicular adenocarcinoma with clear cells, occurring in infancy. *Cancer,* **9:** 165, 1956.

5 MAGNER, D., CAMPBELL, J. S. and WIGLESWORTH, F. W.: Testicular adenocarcinoma with clear cells occurring in infancy: a distinctive tumour. *Can Med Assoc J,* **86:** 485, 1962.

6 WHITE, C. P.: A case of carcinoma myxomatodes of the testis occurring in infancy. J *Pathol Bact,* **14:** 522, 1910.

7 ABELL, M. R. and HOLTZ, F.: Testicular neoplasms in infants and children. I. Tumors of germ cell origin. *Cancer,* **16:** 965, 1963.

8 PIERCE, G. B., BULLOCK, W. K. and HUNTINGTON, R. W., Jr.: Yolk sac tumors of the testis. *Cancer,* **25:** 644, 1970.

9 TEOH, T. B., STEWARD, J. K. and WILLIS, R. A.: The distinctive adenocarcinoma of the infant's testis: an account of 15 cases. *J Pathol Bact,* **80:** 147, 1960.

10 HUNTINGTON, R. W., Jr., MORGENSTERN, N. L., SARGENT, J. A., GIEM, R. N., RICHARDS, A. and HANFORD, K. C.: Germinal tumors exhibiting the endodermal sinus pattern of Teilum in young children. *Cancer,* **16:** 34, 1963.

11 HOSER, R., IZANT, R. J., Jr. and PERSKY, L.: Testicular tumors in children. *Am J Surg,* **110:** 876, 1965.

12 DAVIS, A. E.: Rhabdomyosarcoma of the testicle. *J Urol,* **87:** 148, 1962.

13 HOLTZ, F. and ABELL, M. R.: Testicular neoplasms in infants and children. *Cancer,* **16:** 982, 1963.

14 GOWING, N. F. C.: Malignant lymphoma of the testis. *In:* The Pathology of Testicular Tumours. Studies from the Testicular Tumour Panel and Registry of the Pathological Society of Great Britain and Ireland in association with the British Empire Cancer Campaign for Research, edited by D. H. Collins and R. C. B. Pugh, E. & S. Livingstone Ltd., Edinburgh and London, 1965, p.85.

15 MELICOW, M. M.: Classification of tumors of testis: A clinical and pathological study based on 105 primary and 13 secondary cases in adults, and 3 primary and 4 secondary cases in children. *J Urol,* **73:** 547, 1955.

16 WADDELL, R. W.: Testicular lymphoblastomas in children: Report of a case and review of the literature. *J Urol,* **85:** 956, 1961.

17 TURLEY, H. K. and MOORE, T. D.: Malignant lymphoma primarily manifested as a testicular tumor. *J Urol,* **68:** 744, 1952.

18 MILLER, A. L., Jr. and SHARP, L.: Unusual intrascrotal tumors. *J Urol,* **91:** 273, 1964.

19 STOUT, A. P.: Reticulum cell type lymphosarcoma of testis. *In:* Tumor Seminar, conducted by A. P. Stout, San Antonio, 1950. *Tex J Med,* **47:** 575, 1951.

20 THACKRAY, A. C.: Seminoma. *In:* The Pathology of Testicular Tumours. Studies from the Testicular Tumor Panel and Registry of the Pathological Society of Great Britain and Ireland in association with the British Empire Cancer Campaign for Research, edited by D. H. Collins and R. C. B. Pugh, E. & S. Livingstone Ltd., Edinburgh and London, 1965, p. 12.

MANAGEMENT OF EMBRYONAL ADENOCARCINOMA OF THE TESTIS IN CHILDHOOD: AN ANALYSIS OF 164 CASES

ROBERT D. JEFFS, M.D., F.R.C.S.(C)*

"For various reasons, tumors of the testis have always tended to arouse a measure of interest somewhat out of proportion to their clinical frequency. Such tumors are, of course, comparatively rare and few surgeons are given an opportunity for studying a large series at first hand"[1].

Testis tumor, with an incidence of two per 100,000 in boys under 15 years of age, ranks seventh among malignancies of children. Childhood tumors represent 2% to 5% of testicular tumors totalled for all ages[2]. The majority of testis tumors in adults originate in the primitive germ cells but non-germ cell tumors are relatively more frequent in childhood.

Of the 35 testicular tumors identified and treated at the Hospital for Sick Children, Toronto, since 1927, 10 were of non-germ cell origin; 12 were teratomas; and the remaining 13 were embryonal adenocarcinoma. This paper describes current concepts of management of embryonal adenocarcinoma based upon an analysis of 151 cases from the literature, and these 13 cases from the records of the Hospital for Sick Children.

The age at orchidectomy, the treatment and follow-up studies in these 13 patients are listed in Table I. The classification of testis tumors in Table II gives pathological types and stages of involvement.

Embryonal adenocarcinoma of childhood, the pathological type under consideration in this paper, is a separate entity from the embryonal carcinoma, which occurs in adults.

Embryonal adenocarcinoma is characterized by adenomatous, papillary or cystic formations of flattened, cuboidal or columnar cells and mesenchymal component. These undifferentiated tissues cannot be recognized as ectoderm, endoderm or mesoderm[3]. Teilum[4] in 1959 likened the tissue to extraembryonic endoderm of the primitive yolk sac. Magner[5] in 1951, described its distinctive features and called it "testicular adenocarcinoma with clear cells". Teoh[6] in 1960 postulated that the tumor arose from immature tubules of the fetal or infant testis before spermatic or sertoli cells had differentiated. He introduced the name "orchioblastoma". Young[3] states that the term "embryonal adenocarcinoma", as used in his laboratory since 1936, is specific enough to indicate that the tumor differs from adult embryonal carcinoma and yet is malignant.

---

*Chief, Division of Urology, The Hospital for Sick Children, Toronto; and Assistant Professor of Surgery, University of Toronto.

TABLE I

Embryonal Adenocarcinoma
Treated at The Hospital For Sick Children, Toronto
1927 – 1972

Case	Diagnosis Age (mo.)	Orchidectomy	Lymphadenectomy	Radiation	Survival (mo.)	Remarks
1	20	Yes	No	No	D 1/30	Large Tumor (massive retroperitoneal glands)
2	14	”	”	”	D 12	Scrotal involvement. Recurrence 6 mo./glands
3	66	”	Yes – Neg.	”	A 36	
4	66	”	” ”	”	A 15	
5	22	”	No	”	A 60	
6	14	”	”	”	A 180	
7	16	”	”	”	A 72	Extension to epididymis
8	22	”	”	”	A 36	
9	14	”	”	”	A 72	Extension to epididymis
10	9	”	”	Yes (Scrot. & Abd.)	A 228	
11	8	”	Yes – Neg.	No	A 18	
12	18	”	No	Yes (Scrot. Ing. & Abd.)	A 120	Tumor needled for diagnosis
13	3	”	”	No	A 84	

TABLE II

Classification of Testis Tumors

Pathological Type	Pathological Stage
Germ cell tumors:	
1 Seminoma	A Local – confined to testis
2 Embryonal carcinoma	B Regional lymphatic involvement
2a Embryonal adenocarcinoma of childhood	C Distant dissemination
3 Teratoma	
4 Choriocarcinoma	
Non-germ cell tumors:	
1 Gonadal stromal tumors	
2 Paratesticular sarcoma	

Embryonal adenocarcinoma occurs most frequently in children under two years of age but has been seen occasionally in adults. The right and left testes are involved with equal frequency and the tumor presents as a firm, non-tender swelling, which does not transilluminate. Retroperitoneal spread to regional lymph glands is less frequent at diagnosis and the survival rate of 65% is significantly better than in the adult embryonal carcinoma.

Embryonal carcinoma of adults, described by Dixon and Moore[7] is also characterized by undifferentiated epithelial and mesenchymal tissue but the epithelial tissue is less well organized. It is doubtful if embryonal carcinoma exists before puberty[3]. Usually, by the time the diagnosis is made, the tumor has spread to the retroperitoneal glands in 50% of cases and the prognosis approximates 45% survival.

Ideal treatment for embryonal adenocarcinoma in children is not yet clearly established. Orchidectomy, retroperitoneal lymphadenectomy, irradiation and chemotherapy have all been used singly or in combination. The number of cases in most reported series is too small to permit a conclusion about the effect of treatment on the natural history of the disease (Table I). A series collected from the literature would indicate more accurately how the mortality rate is changed by methods of treatment.

Table III lists the authors and the 164 cases selected from their papers tabulated by age, treatment and results.

No attempt was made to review all of the world literature. Patients over 12 years of age at diagnosis were excluded on the basis that the tumor might represent adult embryonal carcinoma. Cases with a follow-up of less than 12 months were excluded because a cure was defined as "alive and well 12 months

TABLE III

Authors	Selected Cases
Abell and Holtz[11]	12
Anderson and Huston[12]	1
Batsakis[13]	1
Bormel and Mays[14]	1
Doyle[15]	1
Dutta-Chaudhuri[16]	1
Gahagan and Gahagan[17]	1
Gangai[18]	1
Gross[19]	8
Hodson and Perez-Mesa[20]	2
Houser *et al.*[8]	1
Huntington[21]	6
Jeffs	13
Johnson *et al.*[2]	4
Kretschmer[22]	1
Kutzmann and Gibson[23]	1
Lewis[24]	1
Magner *et al.*[5]	11
Matsumoto[9]	28
McCullough *et al.*[26]	2
Melicow[27]	1
Meltzer and Bloom[28]	1
Phelan *et al.*[29]	2
Pierce *et al.*[30]	11
Ravich *et al.*[31]	1
Ross and Morrow[32]	1
Rusche[33]	4
Schmid[34]	1
Scobie[35]	4
Sharma and Samuel[36]	1
Silvert[37]	1
Staubitz *et al.*[38]	3
Tefft *et al.*[39]	6
Teoh *et al.*[6]	8
Weitzner[40]	1
Williams[42]	3
Young *et al.*[3]	18
Total	164

after operation", and because most of the patients who died had evidence of metastases within 12 months.

It was assumed that embryonal carcinoma, under the age of 12 years, was the same tumor as embryonal adenocarcinoma[3]. This assumption seems to be confirmed by the finding that cases under two years of age, that Houser *et al.*[8] designated as "embryonal carcinoma", had a 72.4% survival rate, and those he designated "embryonal adenocarcinoma" had a 72% survival rate.

Table IV shows that in the 164 cases, there were 56 deaths – a mortality rate of 35%. The average age of the group was 19.6 months with an age range from one month to 120 months. The cases were grouped according to age with all types of treatment included. The increasing mortality rate with age indicates that the tumor is congenital. The older child is more likely to have metastatic tumor and to require more intensive treatment.

TABLE IV

All Treatments Included

Age (mo.) at Diagnosis	Average Age	No. Cases	No. Dead	Mortality %
0 to 12	8.3	54	8	15
12+ to 24	18.4	76	28	37
24+ to 144	41.9	34	20	59
Total (for series)	19.6	164	56	35

Table V lists the patients who received orchidectomy alone (Treatment A); orchidectomy with radiation to the retroperitoneal glands (Treatment B); and orchidectomy *plus* lymphadenectomy, with or without additional treatment (Treatment C). Six patients treated by orchidectomy and chemotherapy are not included. The data in Table V were analyzed statistically to determine whether there were significant differences between age and treatment groups. The 158 cases analyzed revealed 51 deaths, giving a death rate of 32%.

In Treatment A, 4% mortality in the 0 to 12 months group is significantly lower than expected, and 71% mortality in the 24+ to 144 months group is significantly higher than expected. The 39% mortality rate in Treatment B, totalled for all ages, is as expected but 11% mortality in Treatment C is significantly lower than expected. When divided into the three age groups, comparison of Treatments A, B and C does not demonstrate significant differences because of the small number of cases in some age groups.

TABLE V

Analysis of Treatment

Age (mo.) at Diagnosis	No. Cases	No. Dead	Mortality %
TREATMENT A – Orchidectomy alone			
0 to 12	23	1	4
12+ to 24	40	16	40
24+ to 144	17	12	71
Total	80	29	36 average
TREATMENT B – Orchidectomy and Radiation			
0 to 12	19	4	21
12+ to 24	24	11	46
24+ to 144	8	4	50
Total	51	19	39 average
TREATMENT C – Orchidectomy and Lymphadenectomy			
0 to 12	10	1	10
12+ to 24	10	0	0
24+ to 144	7	2	29
Total	27	3	11 average
Total analyzed	158	51	32 average

This analysis indicates a mortality rate, which increases with age and decreases in patients receiving retroperitoneal lymphadenectomy. There is no significant reduction in mortality when retroperitoneal nodes were irradiated after orchidectomy.

PRIMARY LESION

Data available on size of tumor, duration of symptoms and local extensions were frequently too incomplete to make a statistical analysis in the collected cases. One would expect that large tumors, known to have been present for long periods would have a poor prognosis, yet many patients with large tumors were cured and some patients with small tumors died. Scrotal invasion was a bad prognostic sign but extensions to the epididymis alone did not appear to influence survival. A long period between finding the mass and beginning treatment did not consistently affect the prognosis. Tumor size, duration of symptoms and epididymal invasion did not consistently indicate the need for additional treatment after orchidectomy.

RADIATION

This collected series spans more than 20 years during which time radiation therapy has greatly improved. The results of radiation might have been better if all of the patients had been treated in the past five years. Matsumoto[9] in 1970, presented 19 cases, all under the age of 12 months treated by orchidectomy and irradiation without a death. His results must be compared with those achieved for the 23 patients in the same age group treated by orchidectomy alone, with one death (Table V, Treatment A). Radiation of the retroperitoneal area risks damage to the spinal epiphyses, local growth retardation, and possible damage to the kidney. On the other hand, Young *et al.*[3] report that irradiation cured a patient with pulmonary metastases.

RETROPERITONEAL LYMPHADENECTOMY

The spread of embryonal adenocarcinoma to the retroperitoneal glands in advanced cases has been confirmed at necropsy. Lymphadenectomy cured one patient in whom tumor was found in the retroperitoneal glands. Two patients in whom resected retroperitoneal nodes were free of tumor subsequently died of distant metastases. Young *et al.*[3] described a patient who had pulmonary metastases at the time of orchidectomy but had no evidence of retroperitoneal spread. The reasons for significantly better prognosis in patients treated by lymphadenectomy are obscure. Pathological examination of the nodes removed in 27 patients showed metastatic tumor in one patient only. No deaths from retroperitoneal lymphadenectomy have been reported but the operation must carry some risk. Defective ejaculation[10], which does occur after bilateral dissection, may be permanent.

CHEMOTHERAPY

The effect of various drugs on survival cannot be evaluated because the number of cases reported is small. Chemotherapy for metastatic tumors would be advisable to potentiate the effect of radiation.

MANAGEMENT

An enlarged, painless testicle in a child requires immediate investigation. Fluid in the hydrocele sac does not exclude tumor. Transillumination and comparison of the testes should differentiate between simple hydrocele and testis tumor. Aspiration of the scrotum is contraindicated because it may facilitate local tumor spread.

Preoperative investigation should include an intravenous pyelogram, a metastatic survey and urine tests for chorionic gonadotropins and 17-ketosteroids.

High inguinal orchidectomy, after clamping the cord and before mobilization of the testis for inspection, is the initial treatment. Where possible, funicular lymphangiography, carried out at the same time, or pedal lymphangiography later, may help to determine if lymph nodes are involved. Histopathological examination will determine the type of tumor and degree of local extension.

Knowledge of the pathological stage of the tumor (Table II) directs additional treatment. Clinical and radiological examination cannot clearly indicate if a tumor is confined to the testis (Stage A), or has spread to retroperitoneal glands (Stage B). Evidence of pulmonary and other distant metastases confirm the presence of Stage C disease.

Bilateral retroperitoneal lymphadenectomy provides the opportunity to differentiate pathologically between Stage A and Stage B disease. Table V clearly indicates that this procedure improves prognosis in children over 12 months of age, who have an expected mortality of 44%. In children under 12 months, who have an expected mortality of 15%, the indications are less clear. Unilateral, extraperitoneal, gland dissection on the side of the lesion carries little risk and can be accomplished in the young child with little or no damage to the sympathetic chain thus protecting ejaculatory function. This operation would provide accurate staging in children under 12 months and might help to reduce the 15% mortality rate.

Patients with Stage A tumor, confirmed pathologically by retroperitoneal gland dissection, require monthly examinations and chest x-rays for one year. In the absence of distant metastases no additional treatment is recommended. After the first year, patients are followed for five years but the interval is lengthened between assessments.

Patients with Stage B tumors may be cured by retroperitoneal gland dissection but dissection may miss spread to the lymph nodes beyond the primary lymphatic drainage. Radiation should be given to the retroperitoneal area in a total dosage of 2000 to 3000 rads in four to seven weeks[9] to anticipate such spread.

Patients with Stage C tumor can be cured by aggressive therapy[3]. Demonstrable lesions should be treated by radiation and chemotherapy. Surgical excision, including resection of lung secondaries and retroperitoneal lymphadenectomy, may be used selectively.

SUMMARY

Testicular embryonal adenocarcinoma in childhood is uncommon, thus the individual surgeon's experience with this tumor is limited. A tabulation of collected cases indicates that the tumor is congenital and that the chance of survival decreases as age increases. Statistically, the prognosis is not improved by irradiation of retroperitoneal glands but is improved by retroperitoneal lymphadenectomy. Operative staging by high inguinal orchidectomy and retroperitoneal lymphadenectomy is recommended in the absence of demonstrable distant metastases.

Stage A patients should be carefully followed after node dissection.

Stage B patients should receive irradiation to the retroperitoneal area. Aggressive therapy, including irradiation, chemotherapy and surgery may be successful in Stage C disease.

This and other methods of management of embryonal adenocarcinoma should be constantly re-evaluated in order to assess the impact of treatment on the natural history of this disease.

REFERENCES

1 FERGUSSON, J. D.: Tumours of the Testis. *Br J Urol,* **34:** 407, 1962.

2 JOHNSON, D. E. *et al.:* Testicular tumours in children. *J Urol,* **104:** 940, 1970.

3 YOUNG P. G. *et al.:* Embryonal adenocarcinoma in the prepubertal testis: A clinicopathologic study of 18 cases. *Cancer,* **26:** 1065, 1970.

4 TEILUM, G.: Endodermal sinus tumours of ovary and testis: Comparative morphogenesis of so-called mesonephroma ovarii – (Schiller) and extraembryonic (yolk sac-allantoic) structures of rat's placenta. *Cancer,* **12:** 1092, 1959.

5 MAGNER, D. *et al.:* Testicular adenocarcinoma with clear cells occurring in infancy: A distinctive tumour. *Can Med Assoc J,* **86:** 485, 1962.

6 TEOH, T. B. *et al.:* The distinctive adenocarcinoma of the infant's testis: An account of 15 cases. *J Pathol Bacteriol,* **80:** 147, 1960.

7 DIXON F. J. and MOORE, R. A.: Tumours of the Male Sex Organs. Atlas of Tumour Pathology, VIII, 31b and 32. AFIP, Washington, D.C., 1952.

8 HOUSER, *et al.:* Testicular tumours in children. *Am J Surg,* **110:** 876, 1965.

9 MATSUMOTO, K. *et al.:* Radiation therapy for the embryonal carcinoma of testis in childhood. *J Urol,* **104:** 778, 1970.

10 LEITER, E. and BRENDLER, H.: Loss of ejaculation following bilateral retroperitoneal lymphadenectomy. *J Urol,* **98:** 375, 1967.

11 ABELL, M. R. and HOLTZ, F.: Testicular neoplasms in infants and children. I. Tumours of germ cell origin. *Cancer,* **16:** 965, 1963.

12 ANDERSON R. E. and HUSTON, C. Tumours of the testicle in childhood. *Am J Surg,* **95:** 445, 1958.

13 BATSAKIS, J. G.: Tumours of testis in infancy and childhood. *Arch Pathol,* **72:** 27, 1961.

14 BORMEL, P. and MAYS, H. B.: Testicular tumours in infancy and childhood: Report of two cases. *J Urol,* **86:** 119, 1961.

15 DOYLE, G. B.: Embryonal carcinoma of the testis in an infant. *Br J Urol,* **27:** 287, 1955.

16 DUTTA-CHAUDHURI, R.: Occurrence of carcinoma of the rete-testis in an infant. *Indian J Pediatr,* **23:** 1, 1956.

17 GAHAGAN, H. Q. and GAHAGAN, H. C.: Malignant tumour of testis in infant. *J Urol,* **78:** 435, 1957.

18 GANGAI, M. P.: Testicular neoplasms in an infant. *Cancer,* **22:** 658, 1968.

19 GROSS, R. E.. The Surgery of Infancy and Childhood: Its Principles and Techniques. Philadelphia, W. B. Saunders Co. 1953, p. 486.

20 HODSON, J. M. and PEREZ-MESA, C.: Infantile adenocarcinoma of the testis. *J Urol,* **89:** 706, 1963.

21 HUNTINGTON, R. W. Jr. *et al.:* Germinal cell tumours exhibiting the endodermal sinus pattern of teilum in young children. *Cancer,* **16:** 34, 1963.

22 KRETSCHMER, H. L.: Embryoma of the testicle in a 5-year-old child. *Am J Surg,* **76:** 99, 1948.

23 KUTZMANN, A. A. and GIBSON, T. E.: Malignant tumours of the testicle in children. *Ann Surg,* 78:761, 1923.

24 LEWIS, E. L.: Tumours of the testis in infants. *US Armed Forces Med J,* **8:** 431, 1957.

25 MAGNER, D. and BRYNAT, A. T. S.: Adenocarcinoma of the testis occurring in infants. *Arch Pathol,* **51:** 82, 1951.

26 McCULLOUGH, D. L. *et al.:* Testicular tumours in infants and children: Report of 5 cases and evaluation of different modes of therapy. *J Urol,* **105:** 140, 1971.

27 MELICOW, M. M.: Classification of tumours of testis: A clinical and pathological study based on 105 primary and 13 secondary cases in adults, and 3 primary and 4 secondary cases in children. *J Urol,* **73:** 547, 1955.

28 MELTZER, A. and BLOOM, B.: Malignant testicular neoplasms in infancy: Report of a case with six-year survival. *N Engl J Med,* **237:** 513, 1947.

29 PHELAN, J. T. *et al.:* Testicular tumours in infants and children. *Surg Gynecol Obstet,* **105:** 569, 1957.

30 PIERCE, G. B. *et al.:* Yolk sac tumours of the testis. *Cancer,* **25:** 644, 1970.

31 RAVICH, L. *et al.:* Embryonal carcinoma of testicle in childhood: Review of literature and preservation of two cases. *J Urol,* **96:** 501, 1966.

32 ROSS, M. M. and MORROW, J. W.: Yolk sac carcinoma of the testis. *J Urol,* **108:** 109, 1972.

33 RUSCHE, C.: Twelve cases of testicular tumours occurring during infancy and childhood. *J Pediatr,* **40:** 192, 1952.

34 SCHMID R.: Zur klink der malignen testikel-tumoren um Sauglings und Kindesalter. *Arch Kinderheilkd,* **152:** 71, 1955.

35 SCOBIE, W. G.: Orchioblastoma: Report of six cases. *Br J Urol,* **42:** 332, 1970.

36 SHARMA, G. C. and SAMUEL, K. C.: Embryonal carcinoma of the testis in an infant. *J Indiana State Med Assoc,* **27:** 57, 1956.

37 SILVERT, D.: Embryonal carcinoma of infants and children: Report of two cases. *J Urol,* **78:** 269, 1957.

38 STAUBITZ, W. J. *et al.:* Management of testicular tumours in children. *J Urol,* **94:** 683, 1965.

39 TEFFT, M. *et al.:* Radiotherapeutic management of testicular neoplasms in children. *Radiology,* **88:** 457, 1967.

40 WEITZNER, S.: Adenocarcinoma of infantile testis. *Am J Dis Child,* **108:** 662, 1964.

41 WHITMORE, W. F. Jr.: Some experiences with retroperitoneal node dissection and chemotherapy in the management of testis neoplasms. *Br J Urol,* **34:** 436, 1962.

42 WILLIAMS, I. G.: Cancer in childhood. *Br J Radiol,* **19:** 182, 1946.

MALIGNANT OVARIAN TUMORS IN CHILDREN

SIGMUND H. EIN, M.D., F.R.C.S.(C)*

In the last 50 years, 15 malignant ovarian tumors have been encountered at the Hospital for Sick Children, Toronto. This paper will analyze and report this series.

CLINICAL MATERIAL

The patients ranged in age from seven to 16 years; almost all were older than 10 years. One-third of these girls had had their menarche by the time the ovarian malignancy was discovered. Most had a rather typical clinical history of a week or so of feeling ill with malaise, anorexia, nausea and vomiting, abdominal pain and a large abdominal mass. In every case an ovarian tumor was correctly suspected and, for the most part, it was apparent on clinical grounds that the tumor was probably malignant. The investigations (blood work and radiographs) tended to rule out other abdominal tumors. Several of these girls had paracentesis and the ascitic fluid showed malignant cells. Aortography was done only in the last two patients. Two of these children had endocrine disturbances; one with a choriocarcinoma and the other with a malignant teratoma.

PATHOLOGY

In a previous study of ovarian tumors from the Hospital for Sick Children, Toronto, 15% were malignant[1]. These tumors represented less than 1% of all malignancies seen at this hospital. The pathological classification of the 15 malignant ovarian tumors in this study are listed in Table I.

TABLE I

Malignant Ovarian Tumors – Pathology

Teratoma	5
Papillary adenocarcinoma	3
Dysgerminoma	2
Embryonal cell carcinoma	2
Granulosa cell carcinoma	2
Choriocarcinoma	1

*Staff Surgeon, Division of General Surgery, The Hospital for Sick Children, Toronto.

A malignant teratoma was found in five girls. Three had widespread disease and in them only palliative surgery was performed. One of these teratomas, in which areas of embryonic carcinoma predominated, presented signs and symptoms of endocrine functioning. A fourth girl had a large ovarian teratoma which, when excised, showed questionable malignant changes in undifferentiated areas. She also had 3000 cc of ascitic fluid which contained many suspicious malignant cells and many peritoneal seedings which were not biopsied. She was treated with radiotherapy and actinomycin-D. At the age of 12 years, the fifth girl had a 24 cm. right malignant ovarian teratoma removed; she did well for five months at which time an asymptomatic abdominal mass involving the left ovary was discovered and resected. She subsequently received a course of radiotherapy.

Highly malignant papillary adenocarcinomas were found in three girls who had widespread secondaries at the original operation. In one of these, the diagnosis at laparotomy and biopsy was sarcoma and the true nature of the tumor was revealed only at autopsy.

Two malignant tumors were classified as dysgerminoma. Two girls were discovered to have widespread embryonal cell carcinoma and ascites. Both these tumors were larger than 15 cm. and weighed over 1400 g. each. One had peritoneal seedings, while, in the other, the tumor had infiltrated the bladder.

Two girls had a granulosa-cell carcinoma. One girl had a varied clinical picture, and at operation, the tumor was obviously malignant. A second girl presented with a huge liver and was thought to have a primary liver malignancy. At laparotomy, she had a granulosa-cell carcinoma involving both ovaries with widespread metastases to her liver. Neither girl showed any evidence of hormonal disturbances, as is usually the case with this tumor.

The only truly functioning malignant tumor in our series was the choriocarcinoma. The malignant teratoma that produced endocrine changes must be classified as "pseudoendocrine". This tumor in some clinical ways resembled an endocrine tumor, although it was classified pathologically as a malignant teratoma.

TREATMENT AND RESULTS

The primary and best treatment of malignant ovarian tumors is complete surgical removal, the technique of which varies with the size and location of the mass and its character. The involved ovary was removed along with the tumor and part or all of the fallopian tube. Only palliative operations were undertaken for those with malignant tumors diagnosed late in their course, in whom the lesion was widespread with intraperitoneal seedings and metastases.

Before 1958, malignant dysgerminoma and papillary cystadenocarcinoma were treated with postoperative radiotherapy without improvement. Since 1958, nine girls with malignant ovarian tumors have had postoperative radiotherapy; three have shown some improvement: one child, five months after her original operation, had a second malignant ovarian teratoma which was also removed. She had not received radiotherapy after her first resection but did have after her second operation; whether this influenced her survival – to date, eight years from the original diagnosis, remains to be seen.

A second girl with an ovarian teratoma with probable malignant change, ascites with suspicious malignant cells and peritoneal seedings has remained well two years after postoperative radiotherapy. She recently returned with an asymptomatic pelvic mass and when re-explored, a benign ovarian teratoma from the opposite ovary was found and excised. There were still many peritoneal seedings (both cystic and solid) and some of these were biopsied and described as "poorly differentiated central nervous system tissue and some striated muscle".

A third girl, who was admitted with ascites and peritoneal metastases from a choriocarcinoma operated on elsewhere three years earlier, received radiotherapy, with good temporary palliation with each of her three recurrences for three and one-half years after discovery of her ovarian carcinoma. The remaining six patients showed little response to radiotherapy.

Chemotherapy was used in conjunction with postoperative radiotherapy in five of our more recent cases, but did not improve palliation or survival.

The survival rate in our series is dismal. Of the 15 girls with malignant lesions of the ovary treated in the last 50 years, only four have survived (Table II). One girl with bilateral malignant ovarian teratomas is alive and well eight years after the discovery of her malignancy. She has received radiotherapy. The second girl with malignant ovarian teratoma who survived to this date has now lived for two years since her operation. A girl who had a dysgerminoma removed almost 20 years ago is alive and well without any other form of therapy. The longest survivor is a woman who had an obviously malignant tumor excised almost 40 years ago. This tumor had elements suggestive of granulosa-cell carcinoma. When last seen in 1959, this patient was pregnant.

TABLE II

Malignant Ovarian Tumors
Survivors and Duration of Survival after Diagnosis

	Number	Survival in Years
Teratoma	2	8, 2
Dysgerminoma	1	19
Granulosa cell carcinoma	1	37

The remaining 11 girls with malignant ovarian tumors are all dead. Nine died in less than one year; the other two died two years and three years after discovery of their disease.

DISCUSSION

Ovarian malignancies in childhood fall into two distinct categories: those of early and those of late diagnosis.

Early Diagnosis

Those diagnosed early seemed to be friable, and adherent to, but easily separated from, the surrounding tissues, e.g., ureter, bladder and cul-de-sac. Fifty per cent of such patients will have straw-colored or serosanguinous fluid in the peritoneal space whether or not they have widespread intraperitoneal metastases. The best diagnostic aid seems to be angiography although, in one of our two cases in which this was done, bilateral ovarian malignancy was not recognized probably because these tumors were too small and were overshadowed by the massively involved liver. In almost every case, one could assert on clinical grounds that the tumor was ovarian and malignant. Furthermore, the ultimate prognosis was usually evident from the findings at laparotomy. Where possible we attempted complete local excision of all visible tumor tissue and when this was done, as in three out of four of the survivors in our series, chances for cure were excellent.

The last of these survivors deserves special mention: the microscopic appearance was highly suggestive of malignant teratoma. The pathologist reported that most of the tissue appeared to be fairly well differentiated. However, some tissue appeared to be of neuroectodermal origin and contained accumulations of very primitive-looking cells. It was difficult for him to say, categorically, whether this teratoma had malignant potentiality or not. However, certain areas were quite suspect. At laparotomy, she had widespread peritoneal seedings (not biopsied) and gross ascites with suspicious malignant cells. To date, she has survived two years after operation following radiotherapy and chemotherapy. However, the peritoneal seedings may not have been malignant.

Late Diagnosis

Malignant ovarian tumors diagnosed late in their course showed widespread intraperitoneal seedings and metastases from liver to pelvis. The primary tumor was often adherent and had invaded nearby organs. At operation 11 of our patients had these findings and, in almost all these, we performed only palliative procedures. With the exception of the girl with malignant teratoma (discussed above), every child in this late group died within three years of onset, most never left hospital despite radiotherapy and chemotherapy.

At present there are two controversies re the treatment of malignant ovarian tumors:

First, what should be done with the opposite and apparently normal ovary? (This question also arises in connection with benign ovarian tumors.) We have not saved the ovarian remnant surrounding the tumor, nor have we been splitting open the opposite ovary looking for small bilateral tumors. At a recent meeting of the Children's Cancer Study Group A Surgical Consultants held at the Memorial Hospital for Cancer and Allied Diseases in New York City in October 1972, about one-half of the pediatric surgeons at the meeting were splitting the opposite ovary. Clark and Exelby of the Memorial Hospital were strongly in favor of this approach, asserting that one-third of all benign teratomas were bilateral – if not in the pediatric age range, then certainly in young womanhood. Perhaps if we had used this approach in our patient with the bilateral malignant ovarian teratomas, we would have detected her second ovarian tumor much earlier. However, in our experience this is the only patient, with either a benign or malignant tumor who later developed a second tumor in the opposite ovary. One pediatric surgeon at the Memorial conference reported that a tumor developed in the contralateral ovary *after* he had split it and performed a wedge biopsy! In any event, there seems to be little indication for radical surgical therapy, e.g., panhysterectomy and bilateral salpingo-oophorectomy in the treatment of malignant ovarian disease in childhood. Our small experience with this disease suggests that here radical surgery is excessive and fruitless.

Second, we have no solid data concerning when to use, and when not to use, radiotherapy and chemotherapy in ovarian malignancy; hence the decision in these young patients may be very difficult. Some surgeons believe that all malignant ovarian tumors should receive this form of therapy but most have concluded that radiotherapy and chemotherapy are indicated only when malignant tumors have not been completely removed. In these cases, the objective seems to be only palliation.

SUMMARY

Malignant ovarian tumors in childhood, though uncommon, should be considered in any female child with an abdominal mass. The treatment is prompt surgical removal if possible. These tumors vary greatly in their malignancy, but if removed before spread has taken place, the child's prognosis may be relatively good. Unfortunately, the complete resection is all too infrequent. Radical surgery has no place in this disease, but radiotherapy and chemotherapy may give some palliation.

REFERENCE

1 EIN, S. H., DARTE, J. and STEPHENS, C. A.: Cystic and solid ovarian tumors in children: A 44-year review. *J Pediatr Surg*, 5: 148, 1970.

TUMORS OF THE BRAIN IN INFANCY AND CHILDHOOD

E. BRUCE HENDRICK, M.D., B.Sc.(Med.), F.R.C.S.(C)*

Tumors of the central nervous system, especially those occurring intracranially, are among the most common neoplasms in infancy and childhood. At the Hospital for Sick Children, Toronto, brain tumors represent about 2.5% of all admissions to the neurosurgical division or approximately 50 cases a year.

Brain tumors, particularly in infancy, are a diagnostic problem. The developing brain has a great capacity for adaptation. Mass lesions may reach great size before producing focal or generalized symptoms and signs suggesting the correct diagnosis.

Increasing intracranial pressure or an abnormal increase in head growth in infants, may be the only manifestation of such tumors. The general symptoms of malaise, irritability, clumsiness or even infrequent vomiting may be so varied and uncharacteristic that they may be mistaken for some relatively innocuous illness of childhood. Hence, physicians responsible for child health, should be ever alert to the possibility of an underlying intracranial space-occupying lesion.

Detailed history-taking and physical examination should include questions concerning behavioral and intellectual change. A decrease in school performance or a sudden slowing in attainment of developmental milestones may be the first symptoms of trouble.

Lack of symptoms, particularly in the cerebral hemispheres, is due both to the compensating elasticity of the child's skull with its open sutures and fontanelle, and to the ability of the immature brain to compensate for gradual functional impairment. However, immature brain tissue is also extremely vulnerable so that severe permanent damage may be inflicted within a relatively short time. The abnormalities detected by neurological examination may indicate only the tip of the iceberg. The degree of brain damage may be much more severe.

In children, most brain tumors occur between the ages of four and 10. The small number diagnosed in infants under one year of age probably reflects the difficulty of detecting behavior change and the difficulties of precise and finite neurological examination. Most infants with tumors present first with the diagnosis of hydrocephalus.

The sharp decline in brain tumors after the age of 10 years is difficult to explain unless one postulates that tumors of embryonic cell types, such as

---

*Chief, Division of Neurosurgery, The Hospital for Sick Children, Toronto.

medulloblastoma and craniopharyngioma, have declared themselves at an earlier age. In adolescents the tumor types typical of adults, including metastases, appear; these include meningiomas, malignant gliomas and secondary carcinomas.

Apart from age and site predilection, certain tumors, such as medulloblastoma and ependymoma, are definitely more common in males than in females.

Most authors agree that, among intracranial tumors of childhood, those in the infratentorial area predominate by a ratio of 6:4. This distribution, of course, is the reverse of adults in whom supratentorial lesions are three times more frequent. Surprisingly, our experience contradicts the general impression. At the Hospital for Sick Children, supratentorial tumors in infants and children are as common as infratentorial tumors, perhaps because we have a specialized unit which deals with central nervous lesions in children and has superior pediatric diagnostic facilities, rather than an institution where the major emphasis is on adult treatment.

The "malignancy" of intracranial tumors in childhood cannot be neatly evaluated in terms of the lesion's histological or macroscopic appearance. The biological prognosis depends upon such factors as size and rate of growth, the degree of structural distortion or displacement, the degree of infiltration, the position of the lesion relative to cerebrospinal fluid pathways or neural structures, and the age and general physical status of the small patient.

SUMMARY

If one were asked to compress all relevant factors covering children's brain tumors into a few sentences, they would most likely read like this:

1. Beware of early morning headache and vomiting.
2. Take alarm at sudden cessation or regression of developmental milestones.
3. Be fearful of seizures, particularly focal.
4. Above all listen to whatever mother says with great care!

POSTERIOR THIRD VENTRICLE TUMORS: CLINICAL PRESENTATION AND ROLE OF SURGERY

H. J. HOFFMAN, M.D. and E. B. HENDRICK, M.D.*

Expanding lesions in the pineal region are extremely rare but do occur more commonly in childhood than in adult life. This paper presents our experience with 30 of these mass lesions at the Hospital for Sick Children during the past 40 years.

Mass lesions at the back of the third ventricle invariably lead to obstruction of the aqueduct of Sylvius and the development of hydrocephalus with consequent signs of raised intracranial pressure. In addition, mass lesions in this area produce pressure on adjacent structures with resultant clinical signs. Pressure on the superior colliculus, which lies just below the pineal gland, leads to loss of upward conjugate gaze (Parinaud's syndrome). Pressure on the third nerve nuclei lead to abnormalities of the pupillary reflexes. Pressure on the superior cerebellar vermis leads to ataxia. Pressure on the hypothalmus can produce hypersomnia and diabetes insipidus. In addition, about one-third of the tumors in this region are atypical teratomas of the pineal; these virtually always occur in males and frequently are associated with precocious puberty.

Since 1934, 30 children with known, posterior third-ventricular tumors have been managed at the Hospital for Sick Children. The first case, seen in 1934, received no treatment and the child died of an atypical teratoma of the pineal two months after admission.

A variety of surgical approaches have been described for extirpation of tumors in this region. Walter Dandy[1] described his direct transcallosal approach in 1921. Subsequently, approaches through parietal lobe[2] and under occipital lobe[3] were described. All of these approaches carried a high degree of morbidity and mortality. In 1943, Russell and Sachs[4] noted that, of 32 patients with pineal tumors who had been treated by surgical excision, only three survived the immediate postoperative period – an operative mortality of 90%. In 1948 concerned by this dismal record, Torkildsen[5] recommended that these patients be treated by radiotherapy after inserting a shunt from the lateral ventricle to cisterna magna.

---

*The Hospital for Sick Children, Toronto.

REVIEW OF MANAGEMENT AT THE HOSPITAL FOR SICK CHILDREN, 1946-1972.

In 1946, Keith, at the Hospital for Sick Children, Toronto, exposed these tumors through the frontal lobe approaching them through the foramen of Monro after entering the frontal horn. Over the next eight years, he used this approach in four patients: two had astrocytomas; one, a typical teratoma of the pineal; and one an atypical teratoma of the pineal. A two-year-old child, with a Grade II astrocytoma in this region treated in this fashion without radiotherapy, is still alive but mentally retarded 23 years later. Another child was treated in this way in 1964 without success.

Torkildsen's method has been used at the Hospital for Sick Children in nine patients since 1949. Four of them died in the immediate postoperative period. Of the five survivors, one died 11 years after shunting and radiotherapy. The other four are alive and well, and have survived from four to nine years. One patient was treated with radiation only and died two years later. Of four patients treated by means of a ventriculoperitoneal shunt and radiotherapy, three died within two years. In one patient, a pineoblastoma was approached through parietal lobe in 1964 and then radiated. This particular patient survived six years and then died of his tumor.

In 1965 Suzuki and Iwabuchi[6] reported on 19 patients with pineal tumors treated by Dandy's method; they had only three operative deaths and concluded that such tumors could be excised safely. Following publication of this report, our service at the Hospital for Sick Children adopted a much more aggressive approach to the treatment of pineal tumors. Since 1967, pineal tumors in nine children, aged five weeks to 13 years, have been treated through a direct surgical approach. These cases are described briefly below.

Case Reports

1. In 1967, we examined a 13-year-old boy who had headaches and diabetes insipidus, but no other neurological deficit. Investigation revealed a small calcified mass in the pineal region. Since he had no hydrocephalus we did not do a Torkildsen shunt and instead, encouraged by Suzuki and Iwabuchi's results, we removed the entire tumor through a transcallosal approach. The tumor proved to be a small encapsulated atypical teratoma of pineal (Fig. 1). Because the tumor was malignant, the boy received postoperative radiotherapy. Six years later, he is perfectly well except for diabetes insipidus.

2. A five-year-old boy, admitted with a nine-day history of headache, meningismus, paralysis of upward gaze, left-sided focal seizures and papilledema, was found to have a mass in the pineal region. A left ventriculoperitoneal shunt was inserted and the tumor, a benign teratoma, was totally excised using Dandy's approach. He has been well for the past five years; his only neurological deficit is loss of upward gaze.

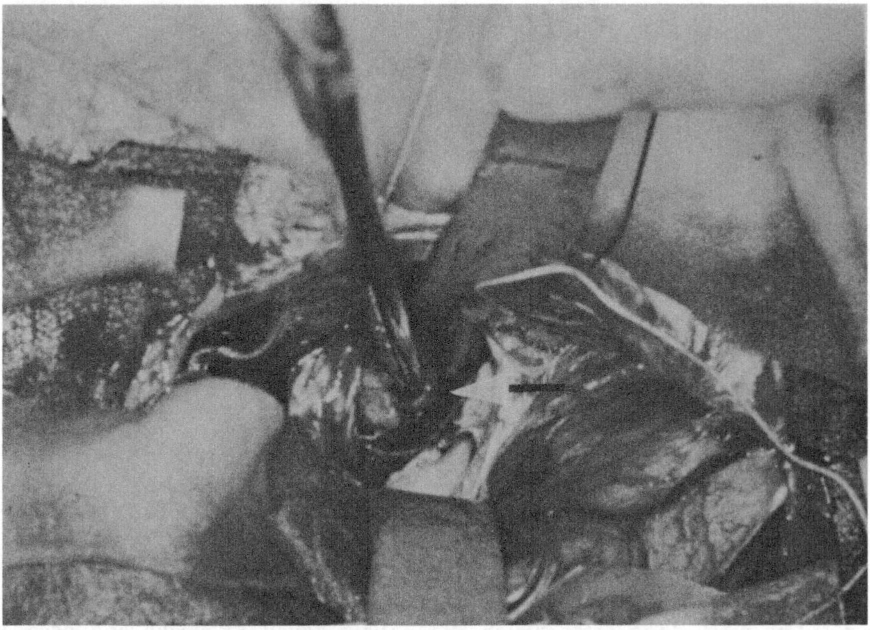

Fig. 1. Operative photograph with arrow overlying corpus callosum and pointing to small tumor in the process of being removed.

3. A 10-year-old boy was admitted to another hospital with an illness which began with lethargy and vomiting. It continued until he was transferred to the Hospital for Sick Children, mute, blind, and quadriparetic. A ventriculoperitoneal shunt was performed for the hydrocephalus produced by a posterior third-ventricular mass but this produced no improvement. Five weeks later, the tumor was partially removed and proved to be an atypical teratoma. Four days after this operation he spoke. However, one month later his shunt blocked, became infected and he died two months after exicision of his tumor.

4. An eight-year-old boy was admitted with a one-month history of headache, vomiting and double vision. He had papilledema, truncal ataxia and VI-nerve weakness. Because investigation showed a pineal mass, a ventriculoperitoneal shunt was inserted, and at craniotomy, an astrocytoma in the pineal region was partially resected. Subsequently, he received a course of radiotherapy. He was re-admitted six weeks later in a deteriorating state and died two weeks later with a massive local recurrence (Fig. 2).

5. A 12-year-old boy with a two-week history of headaches and drowsiness was admitted in a stupor with bilateral papilledema and VI-nerve palsies. Because a ventriculogram, done on the day of admission, showed a mass in the posterior part of the third ventricle, a right ventriculoperitoneal shunt was inserted. His level of consciousness improved. Six days after admission, angiography and an

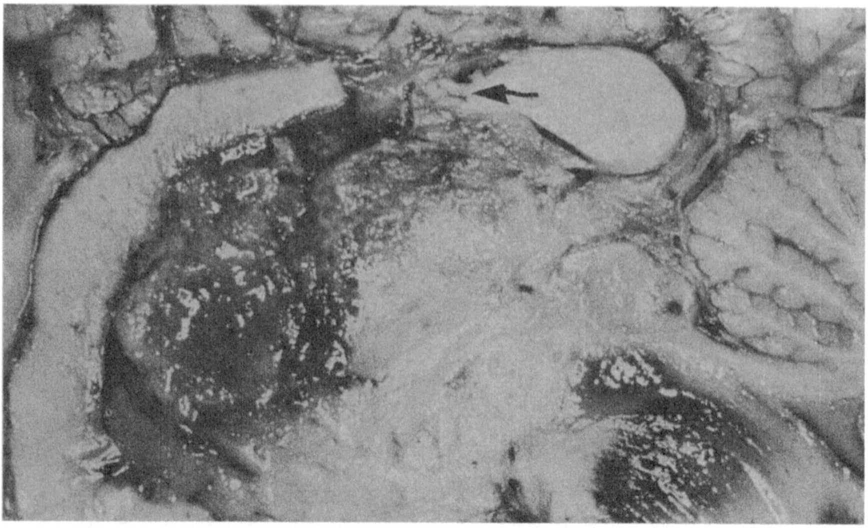

Fig. 2. **Brain of patient with massive recurrent third ventricle astrocytoma which shows (arrow) the operative incision in corpus callosum.**

air study were done after which the patient failed to awake and became decerebrate. At an emergency craniotomy, a hemorrhagic walnut-sized mass, which proved to be an atypical teratoma, was excised *via* the transcallosal route. He subsequently improved but one year later died of tumor recurrence.

Collicular plate cysts, rare lesions in the posterior third-ventricular region, are lined by ependyma or arachnoid and enlarge because of a one-way flow of cerebrospinal fluid into them. Fig. 3, the brain of an infant who died in her crib, shows the massive compression of mid-brain caused by these cysts.

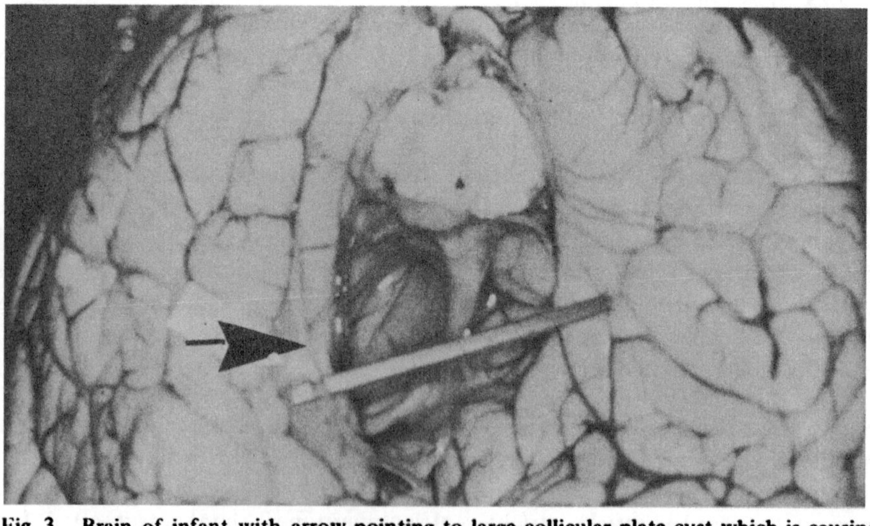

Fig. 3. **Brain of infant with arrow pointing to large collicular plate cyst which is causing massive compression of midbrain.**

6. An eight-year-old girl presented with a long history of school problems and a recent history of headaches and vomiting. She had papilledema, "cracked-pot" resonance of her skull, a right hemiparesis and left intention tremor. An air study revealed a large collicular plate cyst and hydrocephalus. A ventriculoperitoneal shunt was inserted and two weeks later, using Poppen's suboccipital approach, the cyst was exposed and communication was established with the third ventricle. She is well two years later.

7. A five-and-one-half-week-old infant was admitted because his head was enlarging and his fontanelle bulging. A ventriculogram showed a large collicular plate cyst with hydrocephalus. A ventriculoperitoneal shunt was inserted and, a week later, the cyst was exposed by the right occipital approach and communication established with the suprapineal recess and both cerebellopontine angles. The child continues to do well two and one-half years later.

8. A five-year-old boy presented with irritability and signs of raised intracranial pressure. Investigation elsewhere demonstrated a mass lesion in the pineal region. A ventriculoperitoneal shunt was inserted and he was transferred to the Hospital for Sick Children. Here, *via* the transcallosal route, we exposed his lesion which proved to be a benign cyst; a communication was created to the third ventricle. He remains well three years later.

9. A four-month-old girl, admitted because of an enlarging head, had a huge mass filling the posterior portion of the third ventricle. By Dandy's approach, we exposed this large cyst and created a communication between it and the third ventricle. The child has had an uneventful course and now, at age 2½, is developing normally, and has no neurological deficit.

CONCLUSIONS

Since 1967, we have adopted a much more vigorous approach to mass lesions in the posterior third-ventricular region (Tables I and II). We have operatively exposed nine mass lesions in this area with no mortality and/or significant morbidity. Seven of these were exposed by Dandy's transcallosal route and two by the posterior approach. Of these nine cases, four had benign cysts and all of these have been cured. Of the remaining five, one had a typical teratoma and he remains well four years after surgery. One was our original child with the small atypical teratoma who remains well six years later. The other three, two with atypical teratomas and one with a malignant astrocytoma, have all succumbed to their disease. With the modern methods of dealing with cerebral edema and hydrocephalus, the surgical approach to the pineal region is fraught with little hazard and carries a low morbidity and virtually no mortality. The benign tumors, cysts and thrombosed aneurysms of the vein of Galen[7] are curable lesions which obviously benefit from the surgical approach and would not respond to blind radiotherapy.

TABLE I

Methods of Treatment in 30 Children with Posterior Third Ventricle Tumors

Method of Treatment	Period	No. of Patients	Results
No treatment	1934	1	Died in 2 mo.
Transfrontal and shunt	1946-1964	5	1 survivor 23 yr.
Torkildsen shunt	1952-1964	9	4 survivors (1 died after 11 yr.)
Van Wagenen and radiotherapy	1964	1	Survived 6 yr.
Radiation only	1964	1	Survived 2 yr.
Ventriculo-parietal shunt only and radiotherapy	1966-1970	4	1 survived 4 yr.
Transcallosal	1967-1971	7 (6 V-P shunt 5 radiotherapy)	4 survivors alive and well
Suboccipital and V-P shunt	1970-1971	2	2 survivors alive and well

TABLE II

Pathology in 30 Posterior Third Ventricle Tumors

Category	Entire Group	Survivors
Unknown	8	4
Teratoma:		
Benign	2	1
Malignant	1	–
Chorionepithelioma	1	–
Atypical teratoma	6	1
Pineoblastoma	1	–
Medulloblastoma	2	1
Astrocytoma	5	1
Cyst	4	4

SUMMARY

We have abandoned our old approach of Torkildsen shunt and radiotherapy for posterior third-ventricular mass lesions. Instead we approach these tumors directly either through the corpus callosum or underneath the occipital lobe in an attempt to remove them. Tumors are only radiated if histologically they prove to be malignant.

REFERENCES

1 DANDY, W.: An operation for the removal of pineal tumors. *Surg Gynecol Obstet,* **33:** 113, 1921.

2 VAN WAGENEN, W. P.: A surgical approach for the removal of certain pineal tumors. *Surg Gynec Obstet,* **53:** 216, 1931.

3 POPPEN, J. L.: The right occipital approach to a pinealoma. *J Neurosurg,* **25:** 706, 1966.

4 RUSSELL, W. O. and SACHS, E., Pinealoma: Clinicopathologic study of seven cases with a review of the literature. *Arch Pathol,* **35:** 869, 1943.

5 TORKILDSEN, A: Should extirpation be attempted in cases of neoplasm in or near the third ventricle of the brain. *J Neurosurg,* **5:** 249, 1948.

6 SUZUKI, J. and IWABUCHI, T.: Surgical removal of pineal tumours. *J Neurosurg,* **23:** 565, 1965.

7 WEIR, B. K. A., ALLEN, P. B. R. and MILLER, J. D. R.: Excision of thrombosed vein of Galen aneurysm in an infant. *J Neurosurg,* **29:** 619, 1968.

NEURORADIOLOGY OF POSTERIOR THIRD VENTRICLE TUMORS

DEREK HARWOOD-NASH, M.B., Ch.B., F.R.C.P.(C)*

As a rule, posterior third ventricle tumors present with intraventricular obstructive hydrocephalus, the obstruction being at the junction of the aqueduct and the third ventricle. In a slow-growing neoplasm the sutures may separate, giving rise to long interdigitated sutures, whereas in a rapidly growing tumor there is wide separation with short interdigitations. The "split" sutures have no specific characteristics which indicate the site of obstruction in the ventricular system.

The significance of calcifications seen on a plain skull roentgenograph will be dealt with later.

It is our practice to start the investigation with an air ventriculogram and to add pantopaque initially or during the procedure if necessary. This study should be followed by at least a carotid arteriogram *and* a vertebral arteriogram. Brachial arteriography has no place in children, because angiography must be performed by percutaneous selective catheterization via the femoral artery. Great care must be taken to obtain a good venous angiogram in order to outline the deep draining veins in the region of the posterior third ventricle. Radiographic magnification studies with subtraction is part of our routine angiographic technique. Subtraction is often necessary to detect faint filling of the deep venous system which is due to partial occlusion of the vessels by compression or involvement, rather than to insufficient dye.

The radiological diagnosis of posterior third ventricle tumors is often difficult, and numerous special techniques are necessary to establish their character, extent and possible pathology.

These techniques will demonstrate:

Site – Air and/or positive contrast ventriculography and/or cerebral angiography.

Extent – A combination of air or positive-contrast studies and the arterial and venous phases of cerebral angiography.

*Assistant Professor of Radiology, University of Toronto; Pediatric Neuroradiologist, The Hospital for Sick Children, Toronto.

Character – Calcification can be assessed by standard skull roentgenographs, vascularity by cerebral angiography, and the surface of the neoplasm can be outlined by pneumoencephalography and ventriculography.

Differential Diagnosis – If the mass is a benign cyst, it may fill with air. If it is a vascular varix, it will fill with contrast medium during angiography. The upward or medial extension of a cerebral or posterior-fossa neoplasm can also be detected by a combination of the above procedures.

SITE

The primary mode in neuroradiological investigation is the ventriculogram, which may be combined with positive contrast ventriculogram (Fig. 1). This procedure will establish the site of the lesion by illustrating a deformity at the back of the third ventricle. It will also establish the degree of hydrocephalus and indicate whether the obstruction of the aqueduct and third ventricle is complete or partial. This obstruction is due to distortion of rather than displacement of the aqueduct.

Angiography, in our experience, is more useful as an additional investigation than as the initial procedure.

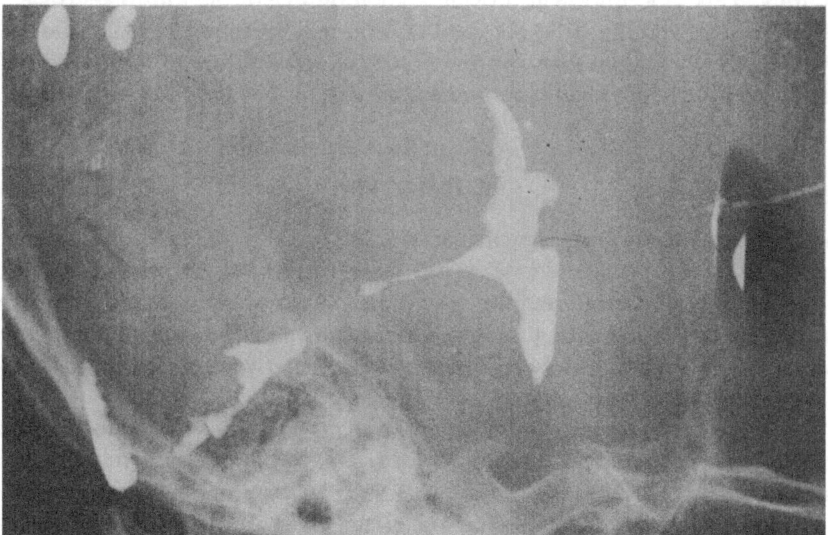

Fig. 1. Positive-contrast ventriculogram showing a pinealoma with an irregular margin.

EXTENT

Ventriculography will reveal only the anterior margin of the tumor. Angiography, both cerebral *and* vertebral, is essential to outline the superior aspect of the lesion. The only way to outline the superior surface is by achieving good opacification of the internal cerebral veins and the vein of Galen. The lateral extension of the mass can be assessed if it displaces the posterior aspect of the basal veins of Rosenthal, posterior choroidal vessels or posterior cerebral arteries, as they course in the region of the collicular cistern. The inferior aspect of the lesion may be outlined by the precentral vein.

It is worth noting in this context that angiography best provides evidence of a posterior fossa neoplasm, such as a medulloblastoma of the superior vermis, which extends up into and presents primarily as a posterior third ventricle mass. Such a tumor produces considerably more displacement of the fourth ventricle and aqueduct than a posterior third-ventricular mass *per se*.

Accurate delineation is most important in assisting the neurosurgeon in his approach and technique. In this regard, it is important to note that the tumor may engulf the internal cerebral veins – a development that is difficult to establish radiologically. Such a tumor is difficult, if not impossible, to remove.

Pneumoencephalography, a dangerous procedure in an obstructive hydrocephalus before ventricular shunting, may be valuable in difficult cases after such shunting. This procedure will provide a good outline of the fourth ventricle and distal aqueduct and the air in the basal cisterns may surround a small tumor.

We advocate aggressive neuroradiological investigation of such lesions and carry out as many procedures as are necessary to outline the mass accurately.

CHARACTER

Air and positive-contrast ventricular studies often provide information concerning the surface characteristics of the mass, i.e., whether it is nodular, smooth or grossly asymmetrical. Before operation, this may help to differentiate a possibly benign lesion with a smooth surface from a malignant-acting lesion with a nodular and irregular surface. However, a preoperative diagnosis based on such evidence may be quite erroneous.

Cerebral angiography with or without magnification helps to determine whether the neoplasm is vascular or not. On the angiogram, neovascularity strongly suggests malignancy – the more vascular the tumor and the greater the flow rate of contrast medium, the higher the grade of malignancy. (Magnification angiography with hyperventilation during anesthesia accents the neovascularity which is unaffected by the resultant low pCO_2.)

Calcification of the posterior third ventricle area in children under 10 years of age, must be considered pathological until proven otherwise. Pineal calcification, which is abnormal in these young children, is commonly seen in teratomas, atypical teratomas and pinealomas.

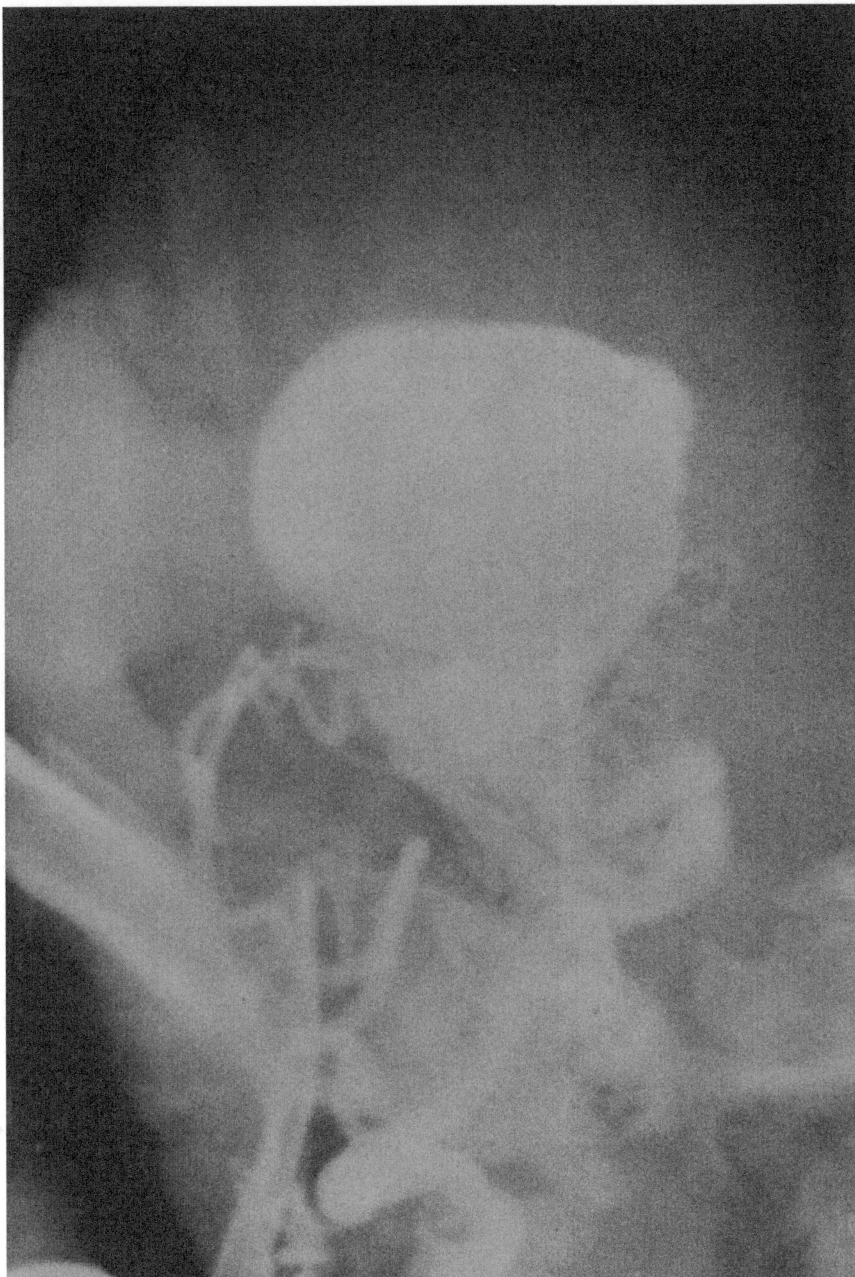

Fig. 2. Selective vertebral angiogram in a newborn showing a huge varix of the vein of Galen with an arteriovenous malformation.

DIFFERENTIAL DIAGNOSIS

Two important abnormalities, which must be considered in the differential diagnosis of posterior third-ventricular neoplasms, are an arteriovenous malformation of the Galenic system associated with a dilated vein of Galen, and arachnoid cysts in the collicular area.

The arteriovenous malformations which present in infancy (Fig. 2) present with severe cardiac failure due to the high blood flow through the malformation. Slow-flow malformations often present about age 2 with aqueduct obstruction and, subsequently, obstructive hydrocephalus. In these cases, a thin crescent of calcification may be seen in the wall of the venous Galenic varix.

Arachnoid cysts in the collicular area may or may not fill with air (Fig. 3), but they elevate the internal cerebral veins and often depress the upper cerebellar veins. Like Galenic varices, they have a smooth outline.

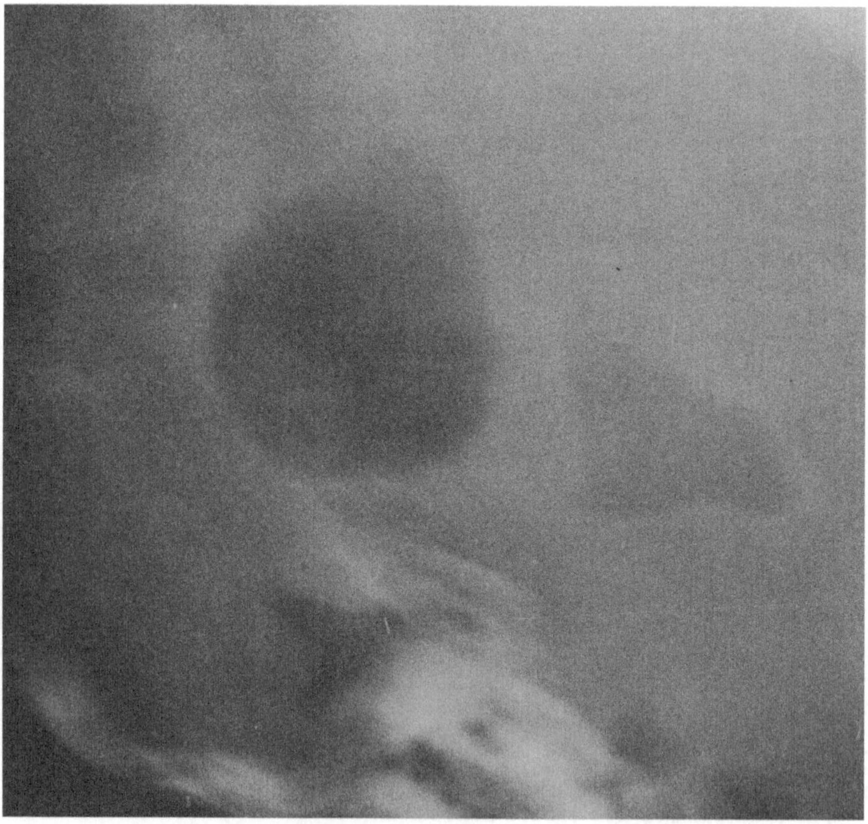

Fig. 3. **Pneumoencephalogram with tomography. A large air-filled collicular cyst has displaced the third and fourth ventricles forward and downward.**

SUMMARY

Neuroradiology, using one or several of the procedures detailed above, will localize mass lesions but in most cases will not suggest an accurate preoperative diagnosis. If neovascularity is demonstrated, the lesion is most probably malignant. Calcification suggests a teratoma or germinoma.

It is possible, therefore, to localize and outline a small lesion in the area of the third ventricle, even when it is exerting only local clinical effects rather than overt hydrocephalus. Anterior, posterior and lateral tomography must be done during the pneumoencephalogram if these small lesions are to be outlined satisfactorily. These special radiographic techniques cannot be done in the majority of radiological departments, yet only these techniques can provide the neurosurgeon with reasonably accurate and satisfactory detail of the lesion. In turn, this information will assist him in the successful treatment of the child with a neoplasm or mass lesion in the region of the posterior third ventricle.

PATHOLOGY OF POSTERIOR THIRD VENTRICLE MASSES

M. G. NORMAN, M.D.*

Reports of 30 posterior third ventricle masses were found in the Tumor Registry of the Hospital for Sick Children. In 21 of these, tissue was available for review.

Of these 30 masses, three were collicular plate cysts. These cysts have a lining of cuboidal cells which may be single or multilayered, and this lining rests on a loose fibrous stroma.

Eighteen were tumors (Table I). The largest single group were the germinomas of the pineal (atypical teratoma of the pineal, "pinealoma"). In five of these, the diagnosis was made from biopsy material, while the sixth was diagnosed at necropsy. This tumor has been the subject of some controversy. Microscopically, it resembles seminoma of the testis and dysgerminoma of the ovary, being composed of large, rather polygonal cells with a distinct cell membrane, clear or scant eosinophilic cytoplasm, a large nucleus and large nucleolus (Fig. 1). Delicate bands of fibrovascular tissue divide sheets of cells into poorly defined lobules. In addition, there are masses of small cells which are indistinguishable from lymphocytes. Occasionally foreign-body giant cells are also present. Although elements of typical teratoma were not associated with germinoma in our material, such mixtures have been reported, and have led people to place this tumor with the teratomas. Nomenclature has been further confused because tumors of similar microscopic appearance found elsewhere in the midline of the brain and pituitary have been called "ectopic pinealoma".

Among these 30 masses there were two benign and one malignant teratoma. The two benign tumors were diagnosed by surgical biopsy, the malignant lesion at necropsy. Teratomas of this region have the characteristics of teratomas elsewhere in the body. There was one choriocarcinoma. The diagnosis, primary pineal choriocarcinoma, requires careful examination of the testes to exclude a primary tumor arising there. These pineal choriocarcinomas may function; hence, measurement of chorionic gonadotrophins would be helpful in making this diagnosis.

Any tumor in the area of the posterior third ventricle may be associated with precocious puberty or delayed puberty, although the former is more common (Table II). The tumors produce their effects because of their anatomical site, not because they produce hormones – the choriocarcinoma being the exception.

---

*Senior Staff Pathologist, The Hospital for Sick Children, Toronto; Assistant Professor of Pathology, University of Toronto.

TABLE I

Histological Types of Tumors in Posterior Third Ventricle

Teratoma:	
Germinoma (atypical teratoma)	6
Typical	
benign	2
malignant	1
choriocarcinoma	1
Pineal:	
Pineoblastoma	? 1
Pineocytoma	–
Neuroectodermal:	
Malignant astrocytoma	4
Mixed glioma	1
Medulloblastoma	2

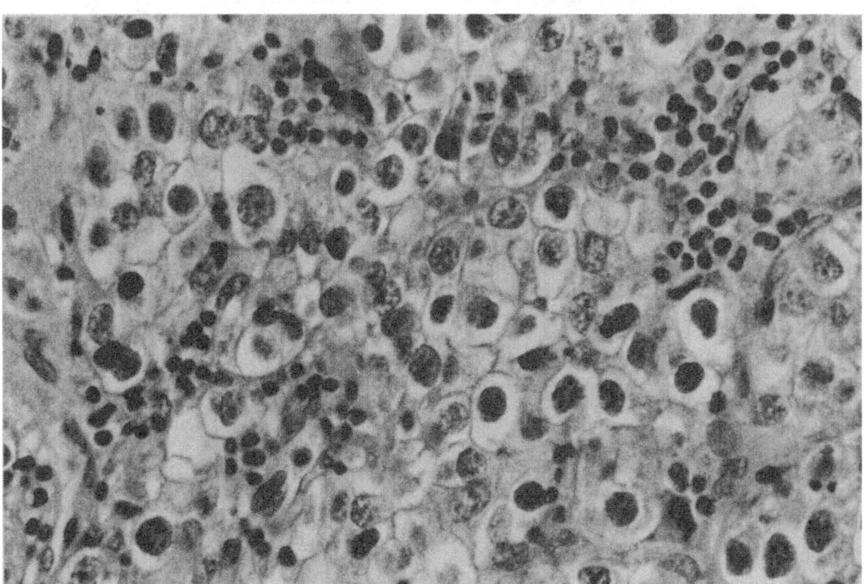

Fig. 1. Germinoma of pineal (hematoxylin and eosin x 250).

TABLE II

Clinical Features Associated with Teratomas of Posterior Third Ventricle

Type	Male	Female	Age (Yr)	Diabetes Insipidus	Sexual Precocity	Signs and Symptoms of Increased Intracranial Pressure
Germinoma*	6	–	9-13	3/5	0/5	5/5
Teratoma**						
Benign	2	–	5-10	0/2	1/2	2/2
Malignant	1	–	16	0/1	0/1	1/1
Choriocarcinoma	1	–	9	0/1	1/1	1/1

*Of three patients treated since 1965, one treated in 1967 and one treated in 1971 by surgical excision and radiation are still living, one died two months after surgical treatment.

**Three of four patients were seen prior to 1960 and died within six months of Torkildson shunting. One patient with a benign teratoma treated in 1968 by surgical excision and radiation is living.

Tumors intrinsic to the pineal are pineoblastoma and pineocytoma. Pineoblastoma is a primitive tumour indistinguishable in its microscopic appearance from medulloblastoma. Our one possible example of pineoblastoma is an extraordinary case (the diagnosis must remain tentative because of the small amount of tissue taken at operation). The child survived some years after biopsy, was treated, and died with two apparently separate tumors – a malignant astrocytoma of the pons and a ganglioglioma of the pineal.

The pineocytoma repeats the lobulated or mosaic pattern of the pineal body, and the cells are arranged in perivascular pseudorosettes or palisades. The nuclei resemble glial nuclei, and cell processes are argyrophilic.

In this series, the biopsy material in four cases was interpreted as malignant astrocytoma, one was a malignant mixed glioma and two were medulloblastomas. Although one of these last might be a pineoblastoma, the tumor was so widespread at necropsy that it was impossible to determine where it had originated. Whether these tumors arose in pineal itself or in adjacent brain is a question which cannot be answered from the microscopic appearance of the biopsy material alone.

Gliomas can be identified at the site of the pineal and, theoretically, astrocytomas could originate in the pineal. Since the pineal is close to ependyma and choroid plexus, the pineal can be replaced by tumors arising in these structures. Not only do pineal tumors present as posterior third ventricle masses, but glial tumors arising in brain can also present as masses in this region.

Chemodectomas and meningiomas have also been found in this region[1], as has an hemangiopericytoma[2].

Cytological examination of cerebrospinal fluid was performed in a number of cases, but generally was not helpful in establishing a diagnosis. If fluid is obtained before any other diagnostic procedure is done which requires needling of the dura, cytological examination may be helpful in the occasional case.

REFERENCES

1 RUSSEL, D. S. and RUBINSTEIN, L. J.: Chapter 7, *In:* Pineal Neoplasms in Pathology of Tumors of the Nervous System, 3rd Edition, Edward Arnold, London, 1971.

2 OLSON, J. R.: Hemangiopericytoma of the pineal body. *J Neurol Neurosurg Psychiatry*, 32: 445, 1969.

RADIOTHERAPY OF POSTERIOR THIRD VENTRICLE TUMORS

R. D. T. JENKIN, M.A., M.B., F.R.C.P.(C), F.F.R.*

In a child with a posterior third ventricle tumor, a decision to treat with irradiation cannot be made until the investigation and the surgical phase of treatment is complete. The children described in this paper, therefore, belong to a select group because not all children survive these initial necessary procedures, nor is every patient then referred for a formal opinion on irradiation.

During the years 1959-1970, 19 children aged 15 years or less presented at the Princess Margaret Hospital with either a "tumor" in the posterior third ventricle region or a proven ectopic germinoma in the suprasellar/hypothalmic region.

Fig. 1 shows the age and sex distribution of these children – four of 19 were aged 7 or less. There were 13 boys and six girls. All 19 were treated by irradiation.

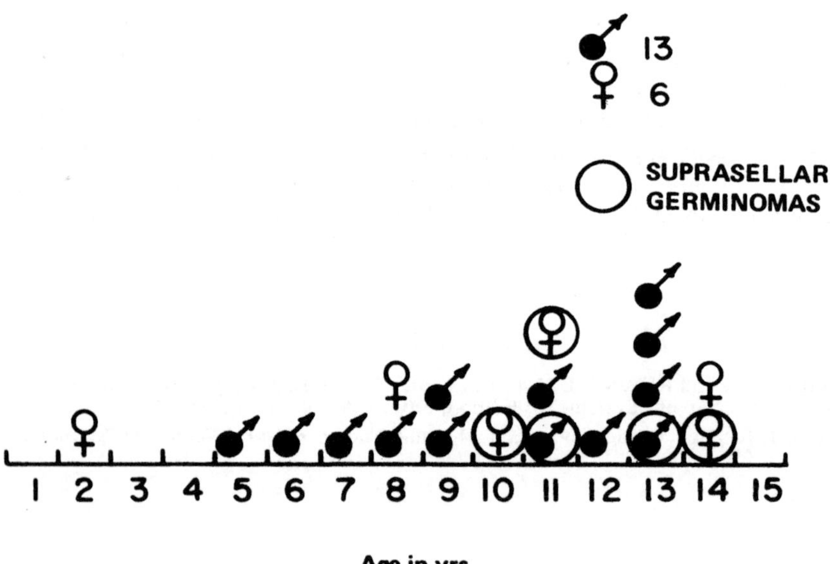

Fig. 1. Posterior third ventricle tumors and suprasellar germinomas. Age and sex incidence in 19 children.

*The Princess Margaret Hospital, Toronto; The Hospital for Sick Children, Toronto; and Assistant Professor of Radiology, University of Toronto, Toronto.

The histological diagnosis was known in only eight (Table I). Germinomas (atypical teratomas) in the suprasellar region are included in this discussion because their radiation treatment is the same as for a germinoma in the pineal region. Indeed these tumors occasionally may represent direct or metastatic spread from a pineal germinoma.

TABLE I

Histological Classification of Tumors in 19 Children
Princess Margaret Hospital 1959-1970

Post 3V tumors	
Germinoma (atypical teratoma)	1
Astrocytoma of pineal (Grade III)	1
"Benign" teratoma	1
No histology	11
	14
Suprasellar germinoma (atypical teratoma)	5
Total	19

No histological diagnosis was made in 11 of 14 of the posterior third ventricle tumors. In these, the diagnosis was based on the clinical picture and neuroradiological investigation alone. Only three of these 14 children did not require a shunt before irradiation and two of these three had an apparently complete excision of the tumor.

The indications for irradiation in these 19 children were as follows:

Posterior Third Ventricle

Eleven, no previous treatment (except shunt).

Three, to supplement apparently complete excision (patients of Dr. H. J. Hoffman):

(a) One, a patient with diabetes insipidus, was irradiated after excision of an encapsulated 2 cm. germinoma of the pineal;

(b) One, after excision of a lemon-sized Grade III astrocytoma in the pineal region;

(c) One, after excision of an apparently benign teratoma of the pineal because the cerebrospinal fluid (CSF) contained abnormal cells of epithelial origin.

Suprasellar Region

Five, germinomas. Previous operative treatment was limited to biopsy or partial excision.

RESULTS

All 19 children completed a course of radical irradiation. Fig. 2 shows their subsequent survival. Five years from diagnosis, 11 of 14 were alive. In October 1972, 11 of this group are alive and eight dead. Of these eight, six died during the first year after diagnosis, and two died eight and 11 years after diagnosis.

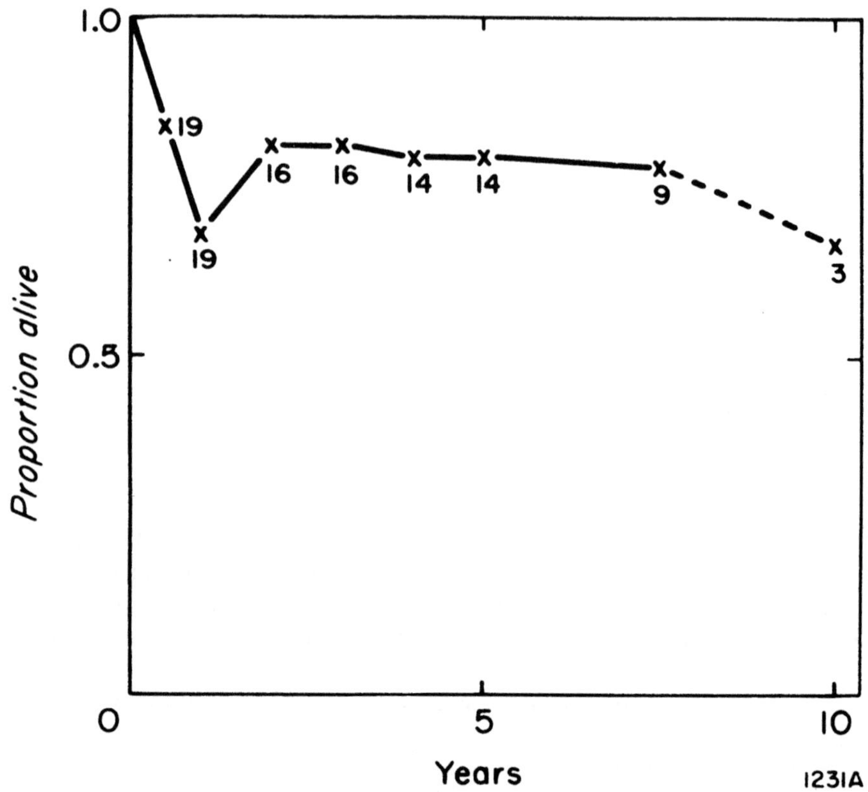

Fig. 2. Posterior third ventricle tumors and suprasellar germinomas. Proportion alive measured from the commencement of irradiation. The numerals indicate the number of children assessible at each point in time.

Certain features of these results are worthy of emphasis:

Ectopic Germinomas

Four of five children with this tumor died within a year of diagnosis. All these children had diabetes insipidus and decreased anterior pituitary function. In addition, four had a variable hypernatremia with inappropriate thirst; these four succumbed during the first year with terminal hypernatremia – an important contributing factor to death. Two of these four underwent autopsy but no residual tumor was found. From this experience, it appears that, irrespective of the degree of tumor control, the lesion destroying or impairing thirst and/or electrolyte control is irreversible. In the time between diagnosis and death, these children lead a hazardous existence; they have highly unstable electrolyte and water control, and endure repeated life-threatening episodes of severe hypernatremia.

Diabetes Insipidus

Seven of these 19 children presented with diabetes insipidus: the four with ectopic germinomas have been described; the remaining three are alive five, eight and 11 years from diagnosis but the diabetes persists. As a general rule, diabetes insipidus is irreversible despite tumor control. If moderate improvement subsequently occurs, the physician should suspect a decrease in anterior pituitary function.

Quality of Life

The survival curve is no more than a limiting parameter in describing subsequent existence. The quality of subsequent life should carry much weight in the initial treatment decision, particularly in the management of brain tumors.

Of the 13 children who survived more than one year from diagnosis, eight are leading reasonably normal lives without major functional impairment. However, five were not so fortunate. Two are retarded and will probably not achieve more than a sheltered workshop type of existence. One is blind but otherwise doing well at a school for the blind. One child had a slow progression of neurological symptoms over several years and died a quadriplegic at eight years of age. The last child required repeated hospital admissions for shunt revisions over an 11-year period after diagnosis and, finally, for the year or two before death was considered to have tumor recurrence.

The final result of irradiation in 19 children may be summed up as follows: eight have done extremely well, five had a marked prolongation of life but with a major handicap, and six were only transiently improved and died during the first year.

Method of Irradiation

Volume. It is clearly established that germinomas and malignant teratomas of the pineal region may occasionally metastasize within the subarachnoid space. For this reason, elective irradiation, either of the whole brain or whole CNS, should be considered in this group of tumors.

When current survival is compared with the volume irradiated (Table II) we see that within the limits of this small series, results were poor only when a small volume was irradiated. After treatment of fields less than 60 $cm.^2$, two of six children lived, compared to any larger volume, after which nine of 13 survived.

TABLE II

Posterior Third Ventricle Tumors and Suprasellar Germinomas Volume Irradiated is Compared with Current Survival

		Local		Local + Whole Brain (7) or C. N. S. (2)
		Small $< 60\ cm^2$	Medium $>60\ cm^2$	
Dead	8	4	1	3
Alive	11	2	3	6

Our data does not permit any conclusions concerning the value of elective whole brain or whole CNS irradiation. Two patients received whole CNS irradiation. An 11-year-old boy, who had an ectopic germinoma and abnormal cells in the CSF, developed a symptomatic, proven spinal cord deposit during the first week of "elective" spinal irradiation. He died with uncertain tumor control and hypernatremia two months later. A 15-year-old boy, who underwent excision of an apparently benign teratoma of the pineal, also had abnormal cells in his CSF, probably of epithelial origin. He remains well four years later.

Our present policy is to treat the primary tumor with opposed fields of not less than 10 x 10 cm. and to electively irradiate the whole brain in children with germinomas, malignant teratomas or if the histology is unknown. Whole CNS irradiation is reserved for the occasional child with abnormal cytology. It may be that a myelogram should be performed routinely in such children to exclude gross but asymptomatic meningeal disease.

In view of the fact that only one child developed spinal metastases among this group of 19, the conservative approach advocated by others[1-3], with regard to spinal irradiation appears reasonable.

Dose. In this series, the dose in the individual patient was that considered to be the maximum safe dose. We have no data concerning the effectiveness of lower doses. Our present practice for the primary tumor, is to give 5000 rads in 28 fractions (5 fractions/week) using parallel opposed 22 MeV beams and a slow start. For electively treated regions of the brain or cord, 3750 to 4000 rads is employed in 20 fractions (5 fractions/week).

SUMMARY

The management of any brain tumor is based on a knowledge of tumor type, that is, a biopsy and, when possible, excision of as much of the tumor as is reasonable in view of postoperative mortality and morbidity. It seems proper that this principle should now be applied in the pineal region. Some children with benign lesions may then be cured by operation and be spared the burden of intensive irradiation.

All malignant lesions should be irradiated, no matter how locally complete the surgical procedure appears to be, because, at this site, irradiation is effective treatment. Recurrence rates following local resection alone will be high, and irradiation given for postoperative recurrence cannot be expected to produce comparable results.

REFERENCES

1 RUBIN, P. and KRAMER, S.: *Radiology*, **85**: 512, 1965.

2 MAIER, J. G. and DEJONG, D.: *Am J Roentgenol Radium Ther Nucl Med*, **99**: 826, 1967.

3 BRADFIELD, J. S. and PEREZ, C. A.: *Radiology*, **103**, 399, 1972.

PANEL ON MANAGEMENT OF BRAIN TUMORS

Moderator: E. B. HENDRICK*
Panelists: D. C. HARWOOD-NASH**, H. J. HOFFMAN†,
R. D. T. JENKIN‡, M. G. NORMAN‡, and M. J. SONLEY††

Dr. Hendrick: To start the discussion I will ask Dr. Sonley whether she believes irradiation of malignant gliomas is worthwhile or should chemotherapy be used?

Dr. Sonley: I think all malignant gliomas should be irradiated.

Dr. Hendrick: What is the value of cerebrospinal fluid cytology in the diagnosis of tumors? In my opinion, it is not very worthwhile. What do you think, Dr. Norman?

Dr. Norman: The yield from CSF cytology is very low. This may be because of poor technique. To be useful, the CSF must be examined as a first procedure, because each time the subarachnoid space is needled, for example, during an air study, a cellular reaction occurs and, on later CSF examination, the cytologist will be confused by odd-looking macrophages. The CSF must be received in the laboratory immediately, preferably warm from the patient. If it is left in the ward refrigerator, cellular detail is rapidly lost. If these criteria are met, we can help, but only occasionally.

Malignant cells can be shed into the CSF only if a tumor involves the subarachnoid space or is at a ventricular surface. Many tumors deep in the brain do not meet this requirement. Moreover, many gliomas are of low-grade malignancy and the individual cells are not obviously malignant, so that even if they are shed into the CSF, the most that can be said is that atypical cells are present. When malignant cells are present it is usually in clinically obvious situations. Medulloblastoma can shed clumps of cells into the CSF. Here, one can make almost a tissue rather than a cytological diagnosis.

Occasionally melanosis of the leptomeninges can be diagnosed. The cells are bland cytologically but contain melanin pigment. Germinoma cells may be characteristic, but I would hesitate to make the diagnosis on that basis alone.

*The Hospital for Sick Children, Toronto.
**The Hospital for Sick Children, Toronto.
†The Hospital for Sick Children, Toronto.
‡The Princess Margaret Hospital, Toronto.
‡The Hospital for Sick Children, Toronto.
††The Princess Margaret Hospital, Toronto.

Cyst fluid from a craniopharyngioma has keratin in it, so that cytological examination restricts the diagnosis to keratin-producing cysts.

Sometimes the surgeon may misunderstand the pathologist's words. In the CSF, we used the expression "atypical" to mean odd cells, e.g., macrophages. It does not mean malignant. If I think cells are malignant, I will say so. Most pathologists do that.

Dr. Hendrick: A question from the audience. Does incision of the corpus callosum interfere with learning in any way? Is there any specific postoperative syndrome?

First, a study was done at the Hospital for Sick Children of children with agenesis of the corpus callosum. No learning disability was found. This was also true of children in whom Dr. Hoffman carried out a surgical approach by way of the corpus callosum.

Dr. Hoffman: There is no specific postoperative syndrome. The main problem is edema of the hemisphere because, in order to approach the corpus callosum, the cerebral hemisphere must be moved away from the falx. Usually a cerebral vein must be sacrificed in order to do this. With steroids and mannitol, one can avoid the postoperative edema which accounted for the high postoperative mortality in the past. We use these agents prophylactically.

Since transient focal signs related to the retracted hemisphere may occasionally be seen, we usually retract the nondominant hemisphere. If hydrocephalus is present and the ventricles are large, there are usually no postoperative signs. The incision in the corpus callosum is small and leads to no ill effects *per se.*

Dr. Hendrick: A question to Dr. Harwood-Nash. In the neuroradiological investigation of brain tumors in children, what is the single most useful procedure?

Dr. Harwood-Nash: This depends on whether the intracranial pressure is elevated or not. I would do an air study either from above or below according to what the neurosurgeon felt was reasonable from the clinical point of view. To take this one step further, if the patient has increased intracranial pressure, then do a ventriculogram followed by a shunt, and then after the shunt, if it was still necessary, do an air study from below. These procedures can be done in any unit. There may be difficulty in getting good angiograms in children but there is no great difficulty in getting good ventriculograms or encephalograms.

Dr. Hendrick: Some neurosurgeons operate on the basis of a radioisotope scan only. Do you consider this a challenge to your territory?

Dr. Harwood-Nash: Not at all. I think it unwise of the neurosurgeon. He is being misdirected!

There is no place at all to operate on any intracranial abnormality on the basis of a scan alone. We use the scan a great deal, as one device in our armamentarium. It is a very good first procedure.

Question: What has been the experience in Canada with systemic chemotherapy, particularly vincristine, in addition to irradiation, in the management of medulloblastoma?

Dr. Sonley: Children with recurrent medulloblastoma usually have a marked improvement with vincristine. While this may initially be dramatic, it usually lasts for only three or four months. Our two longest responses, using maintained therapy, are seven and 24 months. In other recurrent brain tumors the response has been very poor.

Dr. Hendrick: The results of irradiation in the primary treatment of medulloblastoma have been very encouraging over the last 10 years. I have gone through an era when, at first, we expected only four to six months of survival following the diagnosis, whereas now one-half of these children survive for more than five years.

Dr. Wilbur: What has been your experience with the nitrosoureas and intrathecal methotrexate?

Dr. Sonley: We have used BCNU, since it is said to cross the blood brain barrier and to have a response rate as high as 50% in adult glioblastoma multiforme. It is very difficult to quantitate the response to chemotherapy in a recurrent brain tumor; so many have been given dexamethasone (Decadron), or have had a shunt or a shunt revision. Even the measurement of neurological improvement is very subjective. We have seen several recurrent medulloblastomas respond to BCNU, but have been very disappointed with the response in other gliomas. A boy with a brain-stem tumor was maintained on BCNU for two years and has liver toxicity as a result. He was the only child with a brain-stem tumor who responded well and, in retrospect, it is difficult to be sure that he had recurrence rather than a temporarily blocked shunt. Indeed, he demonstrates very well the difficulty in measuring response in these "recurrent" patients.

Dr. Hendrick: What are the relative indications for irradiation or chemotherapy for recurrent tumors? It is often a difficult decision in the individual child.

Dr. Jenkin: If something further than the surgical resection is necessary in the primary treatment of a child with a brain tumor, I believe a radical course of irradiation always is indicated. Except for special studies, we have given this without elective chemotherapy. The value of such irradiation is clear in that an appreciable five-year survival rate is obtained for each tumor type at a level characteristic of each tumor.

As a corollary of this policy, since brain tumors usually recur at the primary site, this will usually be within a previously heavily irradiated volume.

I have been reluctant to re-irradiate during the first year of follow-up, because a second response will be of shorter duration and will be obtained at a considerable risk of radionecrosis. Tumor response to low-dose irradiation is poor, and the initial treatment has usually been taken to a dose of about 5000 rads in five weeks. This remains very much an individual decision depending on the nature of the tumor, the symptoms, the age of the child, and parental attitude. There may be a surgical alternative. We believe re-irradiation is always indicated for late recurrence. The response rate is high and usually worthwhile.

As an extreme example, we would re-irradiate the whole central nervous system in a child with medulloblastoma recurrent two years after diagnosis. Chemotherapy alone has generally been disappointing in children with recurrent tumors and remains investigational. The response rate to re-irradiation is substantially higher than to drug treatment alone, and for this reason, if treatment for a first recurrence is indicated, this will almost always include irradiation. We have combined irradiation with vincristine and BCNU in some children with recurrent tumors, but not in sufficient number to determine whether it improves our results.

Dr. Schweisguth: What are Dr. Sonley's criteria for a 50% improvement on chemotherapy – are they objective or subjective?

Dr. Sonley: It is very difficult to assess response objectively. While we record improvement in each neurological symptom, this alone is not an adequate description. Nervous-tissue dysfunction is not always reversible even if a tumor is controlled. Subjective assessment, both on the part of the child, the parents and the clinician remain very important. The guidelines, which should be used to chart improvement in these children, remain poorly defined.

Dr. Hendrick: This has to be the clinical judgment of several people. For example, I always think my brain tumors do better than Dr. Hoffman thinks they do. You cannot really be dispassionate with your own patients.

Dr. Schweisguth: What are the indications for exploration and removal of posterior third ventricle tumors? In France our neurosurgeons are reluctant to operate on these tumors.

Dr. Hoffman: In general one always wishes to have a histological diagnosis before radiotherapy, but the posterior third ventricle was a horrendous place to get a histological diagnosis. The operative mortality in 1943 was 90%. Leo Davidoff, one of the fathers of neurosurgery on this continent, gave a scholarly address to the New York Academy of Sciences in 1967 in which he pleaded that one of the principles in the care of patients was first of all to do no harm – a principle first enunciated by Hippocrates. For this reason, he felt that neurosurgeons should not operate on posterior third ventricle tumors. The Japanese demonstrated that one could operate in this region without a high degree of mortality. They were operating on atypical teratomas. Recently they have ceased to attempt total removal of tumors in this area because their results were not appreciably different from irradiating. However, these were atypical teratomas. The point I wish to make is, that in children with undiagnosed mass lesions at this site, some will have cysts, thrombosed aneurisms, benign teratomas, meningiomas or dermoid tumors. If it is a benign process, one is doing a disservice to the patient to irradiate it. Furthermore, just exposing the tumor does not carry a significant morbidity, and we have had no mortality from operative exposure of posterior third ventricle tumors.

Dr. Hendrick: Thank you.

HISTIOCYTOSIS X: PATHOLOGY

J. F. K. MANCER, M.D., B.Sc.(Med.), F.R.C.P.(C)*

At the Hospital for Sick Children, Toronto, the tumor registry contains 140 cases of histiocytosis X for the period 1921 to 1972. In a retrospective study of these cases, I classified them clinically and pathologically to determine factors of prognostic importance. This study also sought evidence for or against the concept that histiocytosis X is a spectrum of disease extending from eosinophilic granuloma to the Letterer-Siwe syndrome.

METHODS

The criteria for inclusion in this study were: (a) histological evidence of histiocytosis X; and (b) a follow-up of at least two years. Ninety-one cases satisfied these criteria.

The Hospital for Sick Children receives the great majority of pediatric admissions for Metropolitan Toronto (population 2.1 million) and acts as a pediatric referral centre for most of the Province of Ontario (population 7.7 million). The maximum age of admitted patients is 18, but many teenagers are treated in adult hospitals in Toronto and Ontario. Since older children usually have solitary lesions and the youngest patients have extensive disease mainly, these admission practices would tend to decrease the numbers of solitary eosinophilic granuloma in this series in proportion to more extensive disease. Another factor producing the same effect in this study is the exclusion of many children with solitary eosinophilic granuloma because of lack of follow-up.

RESULTS

Tables I, II and III classify the clinical and pathological data.

PATHOLOGICAL FINDINGS

The histiocytes, which form the basis of these lesions, appear histologically benign, although in some cases there is considerable nuclear atypia. The appearance of the cytoplasm varies with the duration of the lesion. The histiocytes are functionally active and the cytoplasm may contain ingested lipids, hemosiderin, bile pigments and red blood cells.

*Department of Pathology, The Hospital for Sick Children, Toronto, Ontario.

TABLE I

Histiocytosis X: Incidence, Clinical and Pathological Data (91 Cases)

CLASSIFICATION OF PATIENTS	No. of Cases	Males	Females	Age Range at Presentation (yr)	Average Age at Presentation (yr)	Autopsy	Lytic Bone Lesions	Diabetes Insipidus	Exophthalmos	Anemia at Presentation	Biliary Cirrhosis
A. SURVIVORS:											
1. Skeletal involvement only											
(a) Solitary eosinophilic granuloma	32	17	15	8/12 – 13	5.7	–	32	–	–		
(b) Multiple eosinophilic granuloma	23	14	9	8/12 – 8-10/12	3.5	–	23	–	1*		
2. With extraskeletal lesions											
(a) Bone lesions + diabetes insipidus (Hand-Schüller-Christian)	7	5	2	1-7/12 – 5-1/12	2.9	–	7	7	1		
(b) Other systems + bone (unclassifiable)	11	7	4	6/12 – 8-1/12	2.4	–	10	5	1		
B. FATAL CASES:											
1. Slowly progressive (unclassifiable)	12	9	3	3/12 – 10-10/12	1.9	10	9	3	2	–	5**
2. Rapidly progressive (Letterer-Siwe)	6	1	5	4/12 – 1-2/12	0.7	6	–	–	–	5	4

*Considered as involvement of tissue adjacent to a bone lesion and not as a separate site of involvement.

**One of these cases was not autopsied, but was included here because of biochemical evidence of obstructive jaundice.

TABLE II

Histiocytosis X: Sites of Lytic Lesions in the Skeleton (91 Cases)

CLASSIFICATION OF PATIENTS	Skull	Orbit	Innominate Bone	Femur	Ribs	Humerus	Mandible	Tibia	Vertebra	Clavicle	Scapula	Fibula	Sternum	Radius	Metacarpal
A. SURVIVORS:															
1. Skeletal involvement only															
(a) Solitary eosinophilic granuloma	10	3	3	4	1	2	–	2	4	2	–	–	–	1	–
(b) Multiple eosinophilic granuloma	18	2	10	8	4	4	1	3	2	3	3	1	1	–	1
2. With extraskeletal lesions															
(a) Bone lesions + diabetes insipidus (Hand-Schüller-Christian)	5	3	4	–	1	–	1	–	–	–	–	–	–	–	–
(b) Other systems + bone (unclassifiable)	9	1	3	1	1	1	3	1	–	–	–	–	–	–	–
B. FATAL CASES:															
1. Slowly progressive (unclassifiable)	7	2	3	4	1	–	2	1	1	–	–	1	–	–	–
2. Rapidly progressive (Letterer-Siwe)	–	–	–	–	–	–	–	–	–	–	–	–	–	–	–
Total	49	11	23	17	8	7	7	7	7	5	3	2	1	1	1

TABLE III

Histiocytosis X: Sites of Diffuse Histiocytic Infiltration Proved by Biopsy or Autopsy (91 Cases)

CLASSIFICATION OF PATIENTS	Bone Marrow	Neurohypophysis	Periosteum of Sella	Skin	Gingiva	Lymph Nodes	Extrahepatic Bile Ducts	Intrahepatic Bile Ducts	Liver Lobules	Lobules + Portal Areas	Lung	Thymus	Spleen	Endocardium	Connective Tissue	Tonsil	Choroid Plexus	Thyroid	Parathyroid
A. SURVIVORS:																			
1. Skeletal involvement only																			
(a) Solitary eosinophilic granuloma																			
(b) Multiple eosinophilic granuloma																			
2. With extraskeletal lesions																			
(a) Bone lesions + diabetes insipidus (Hand-Schüller Christian)					2*														
(b) Other systems + bone (unclassifiable)				7	–	2													
B. FATAL CASES:																			
1. Slowly progressive (unclassifiable)	5	2	2**	10	1*	8	3	4	1	1	6	5	2	–	2	1	1	1	1
2. Rapidly progressive (Letterer-Siwe)	3	1	3	6	–	5	–	5	3	1	4	6	5	1	1	–	–	–	–

*Considered as involvement of tissue adjacent to a bone lesion and not as a separate site of involvement.
**One case of diabetes insipidus had infiltration of the periosteum of the sella only.

The skeletal lesions tend to involve the larger bones in the following order of frequency: skull, innominate bone, femur, ribs, vertebrae, tibia, humerus, and mandible (Table II). This distribution applies whether the lesions are single or multiple and whether or not the disease involves extraskeletal tissues.

Eosinophilic Granuloma

The typical eosinophilic granuloma (Fig. 1) is a lytic bone lesion composed of loosely and irregularly arranged histiocytes accompanied by variable amounts of an infiltrate, made up of eosinophils and neutrophils in varying proportions. Dense accumulations of eosinophils may be present in some regions, giving the appearance of the "eosinophil micro-abscess". Lymphocytes, plasma cells and multinucleated giant cells may also be found, usually in small amounts. Blood vessels, similar to those of granulation tissue, are usually evident in the lesion. Some eosinophilic granulomas contain foci of hemorrhage and necrosis. Fat stains reveal small globules of extracellular lipid. In the histiocytes, the amount of cytoplasm is usually large relative to the size of the nucleus and the cytoplasm is eosinophilic in hematoxylin and eosin preparations. The nucleus is peripheral and usually kidney-shaped, indented near the centre of the cell. Sometimes there is a moderate amount of nuclear hyperchromatism, but the nuclei do not have enough atypia to establish a diagnosis of malignancy. Erythrophagocytosis may be present. The histiocytes are sometimes multinucleate.

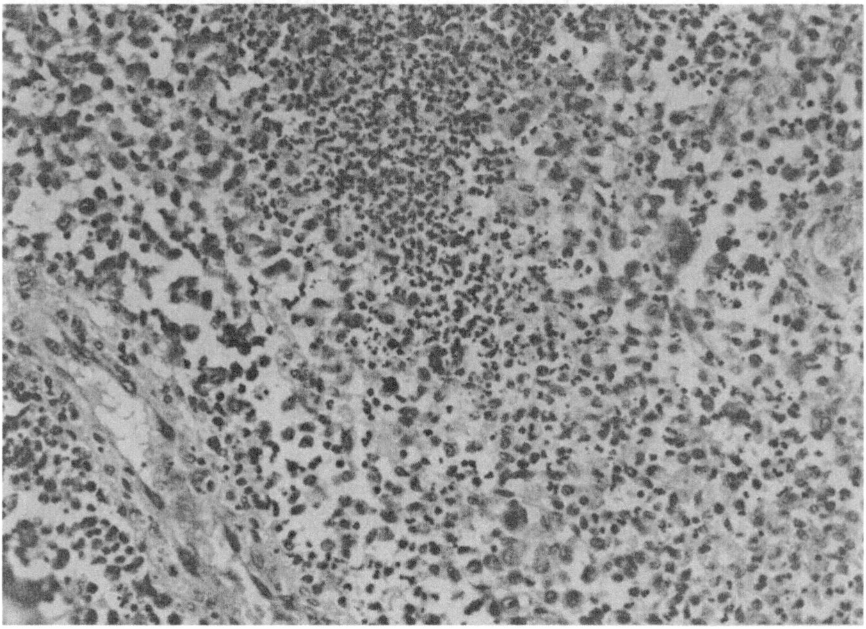

Fig. 1. Eosinophilic granuloma of bone. showing a heavy infiltrate of loosely arranged, non-vacuolated histiocytes with peripheral nuclei. The leukocytic component consists of neutrophils and eosinophils. Note the thin-walled blood vessels passing through the lesion. (x290)

At the periphery the lesion infiltrates for a short distance among the adjacent spicules of bone, where there is considerable osteoclastic activity. The lesion may destroy the cortex of the bone and extend into the soft tissues. When the soft tissue of the orbit is involved, exophthalmos may be evident clinically.

As the lesion ages (Fig. 2), the inflammatory infiltrate becomes less prominent and tends to become lymphocytic. The histiocytes remain and the cytoplasm contains ingested lipid and hemosiderin. Small amounts of fibrous tissue may also be apparent. Otherwise-typical eosinophilic granuloma may present in this later stage of development. Because symptoms occur in the early stage of evolution and biopsy is usually done only at that time, the histological appearance of the later stage of the lesion has not been established with certainty. In this series the only apparent late-stage lesion was that shown in Fig. 3, but since no biopsy was done the lesion may not have been an eosinophilic granuloma initially. Another patient at autopsy had combinations of eosinophilic granuloma, foam cells and fibrosis in single lesions (Fig. 4).

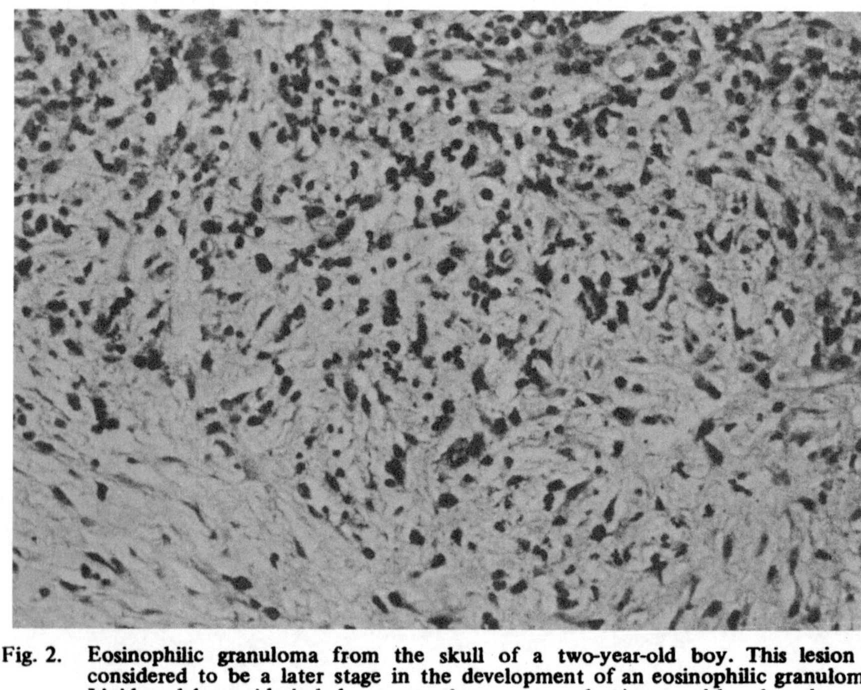

Fig. 2. Eosinophilic granuloma from the skull of a two-year-old boy. This lesion is considered to be a later stage in the development of an eosinophilic granuloma. Lipid and hemosiderin-laden macrophages are predominant, with a lymphocytic infiltrate. (x290)

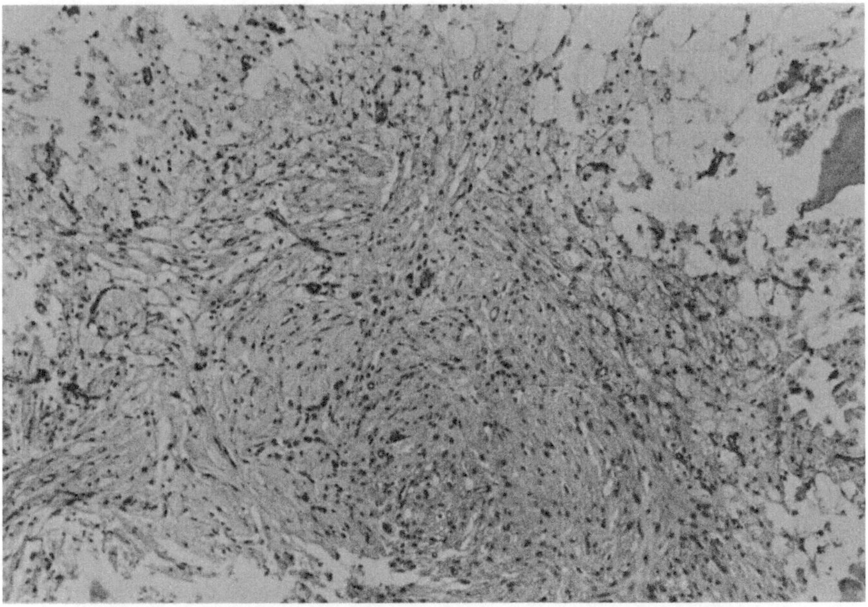

Fig. 3. Probable late stage in the development of an eosinophilic granuloma consisting of foam cells and fibrous tissue. This patient was seen at age five months with a lytic lesion of the tibia, and at eight months she developed biliary cirrhosis secondary to involvement of the biliary tract by histiocytic infiltrates. The tibial lesion was not biopsied but the tissue in this section was removed from the tibial lesion at autopsy (age 19 months). (x115)

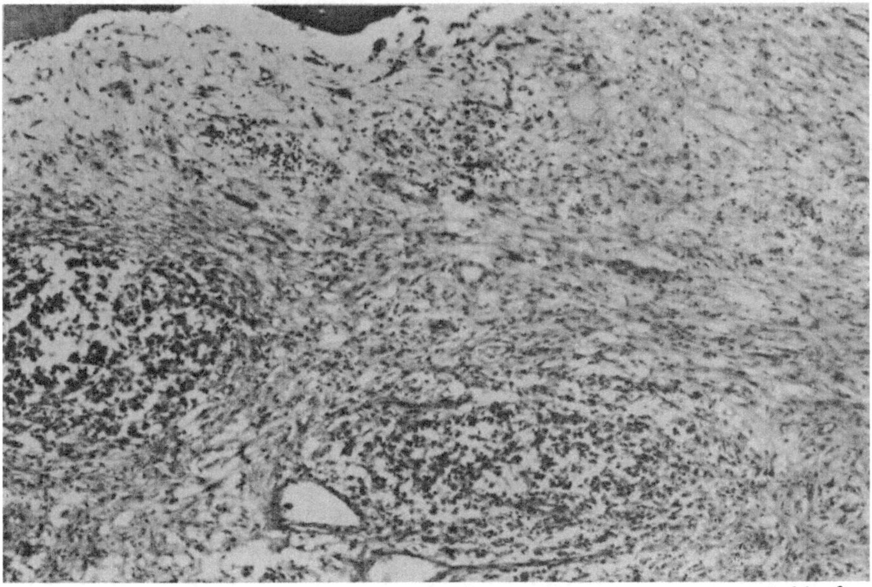

Fig. 4. Lytic bone lesion with large amounts of young fibrous tissue accompanied by foam cells and a lymphocytic infiltrate. The two "granulomatous" areas are composed of non-foamy histiocytes and some eosinophils. (x115)

The rapidly fatal cases of generalized histiocytosis X showed no radiographic and histological evidence of lytic bone lesions. In these patients, bone involvement took the form of diffuse infiltration of the marrow spaces without destruction of the bone spicules. Some cases had a similar type of marrow involvement and also lytic bone lesions.

Extraskeletal Lesions

Most of the pathological data on extraskeletal lesions in histiocytosis X come from fatal cases of generalized disease, which were studied at autopsy. The survivors of generalized histiocytosis X generally were submitted to only one or two biopsies, usually of skin, bone, lymph node or gingiva. No consistent histologic difference was demonstrated between the biopsied lesions in survivors and patients who later died of their disease.

Rapidly fatal cases tended to have massive involvement of many organ systems by loosely arranged histiocytes, which had the same appearance as the early form of eosinophilic granuloma; but eosinophils and neutrophils were not usually present. Some patients had nodular histiocytic infiltrates, which were centrally necrotic, resembling granulomas but consisting purely of histiocytes and containing no blood vessels. The central necrosis was considered to be due to ischemia. A frequent clinical finding early in the disease, was severe anemia; it was often apparent at presentation. In five of the six rapidly fatal cases, the presenting hemoglobin was between 5.4 and 7.4 g. per 100 ml.

Less rapidly progressive disease often started with infiltrates of non-foamy histiocytes, but usually the lipid-containing histiocyte or foam cell, often multinucleate, eventually became dominant. Eosinophils and neutrophils were not apparent at the time of autopsy, except in skin and gingival lesions. These lesions were often ulcerated, which caused difficulty in the interpretation of the inflammatory infiltrate.

Most cases that were ultimately fatal showed evidence of generalized histiocytosis X from the time of onset. Survivors with generalized disease were generally older and had less extensive disease at presentation (Tables I and III). They usually presented with a bone lesion, single or multiple, and later developed such complications as diabetes insipidus, exophthalmos, skin rash or radiographic evidence of pulmonary infiltration. Gradually the disease became inactive and the patient was left with such sequelae as diabetes insipidus.

LESIONS OF SPECIFIC ORGANS

Pituitary

Tissue was obtained only at autopsy. The most consistent finding was an infiltrate of foamy histiocytes in the periosteum of the sella turcica (Fig. 5). One patient who had clinical evidence of diabetes insipidus, had periosteal infiltration alone, without hypophyseal involvement. Most cases of diabetes insipidus had histiocytic infiltrates in the neurohypophysis (Fig. 6). The adenohypophysis was infiltrated slightly in only one case and that patient had a heavy infiltrate in the neurohypophysis.

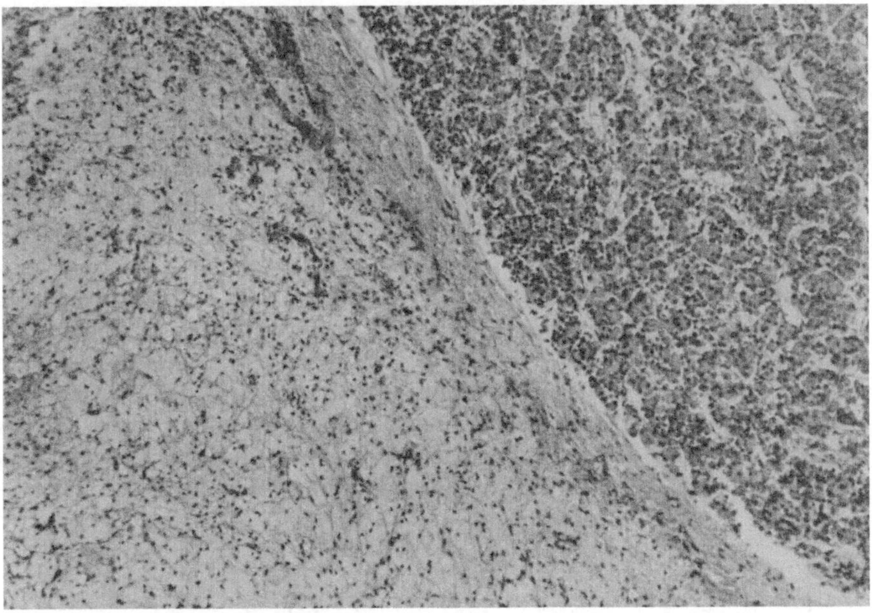

Fig. 5. Heavy infiltrate of foam cells in the periosteum of the sella turcica. The adenohypophysis is not invaded. Such a lesion was usually accompanied by direct invasion of the neurohypophysis. (x115)

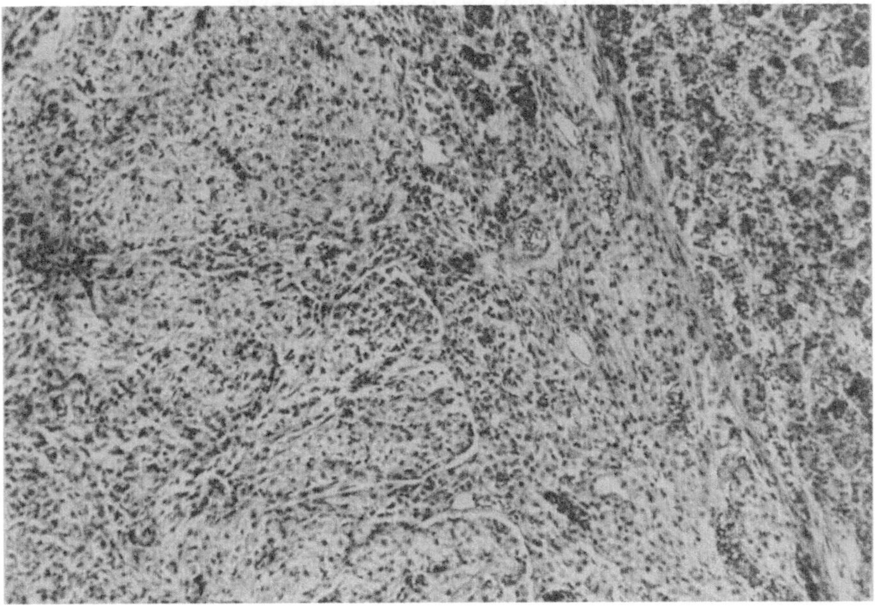

Fig. 6. Neurohypophysis, which occupies most of this picture, heavily infiltrated by histiocytes. The adenohypophysis shows no infiltration. Same case as Fig. 5. (x115)

In the group of survivors, some patients recovered from proved diabetes insipidus, losing their dependence on pitressin.

Liver

Biliary cirrhosis (Figs. 7 and 8) was frequent in the fatal cases, but none of the survivors had any evidence of cirrhosis except one who had received methotrexate and had histological evidence of the type of cirrhosis associated with methotrexate toxicity.

Biliary cirrhosis was considered to be secondary to infiltration and focal destruction of the biliary system. In some cases the obstructive lesion was extrahepatic – at the level of the hepatic ducts or bile duct. In others, the portal triad or intrahepatic bile ducts were involved. Extension of the infiltrates into liver lobules or isolated histiocytic infiltration of the lobular tissue was less frequent. In rapidly progressive histiocytosis X, biliary cirrhosis, though present, was less well developed than in the more slowly progressive cases.

Skin

The presenting complaint in many of the rapidly progressive cases was a skin rash. The rashes tended to become extensive and hemorrhagic, often with ulceration.

A few of the non-fatal cases presented with a skin rash. Clinically, this is a scaly papular eruption resembling seborrheic dermatitis. It is often heaviest on the scalp and occasionally remains confined to that region.

The lesions consisted of an infiltrate of loosely arranged non-foamy histiocytes, mainly in the papillary dermis (Fig. 9). In some cases, the adjacent epidermis is infiltrated by the histiocytes. One patient had a tumor due to heavy infiltration extending into the subcutaneous fat.

There were no consistent histological differences between survivors and non-survivors except that the latter had a greater tendency to heavy epidermal infiltration with ulceration. Eosinophils and neutrophils were often absent from lesions in the fatal cases, but the skin infiltrates of survivors usually contained these cells.

Lymph Nodes

The lesions in the lymph nodes ranged from loose accumulations of histiocytes in sinusoids to diffuse infiltrates, which obliterated the normal nodal architecture. Focal, centrally-necrotic infiltrates were present in some rapidly progressive cases and the spleen and bone marrow usually contained similar lesions.

Spleen

The spleen was usually not involved except in the most rapidly fatal cases. Here the infiltrates were usually nodular and centrally necrotic (Fig. 10).

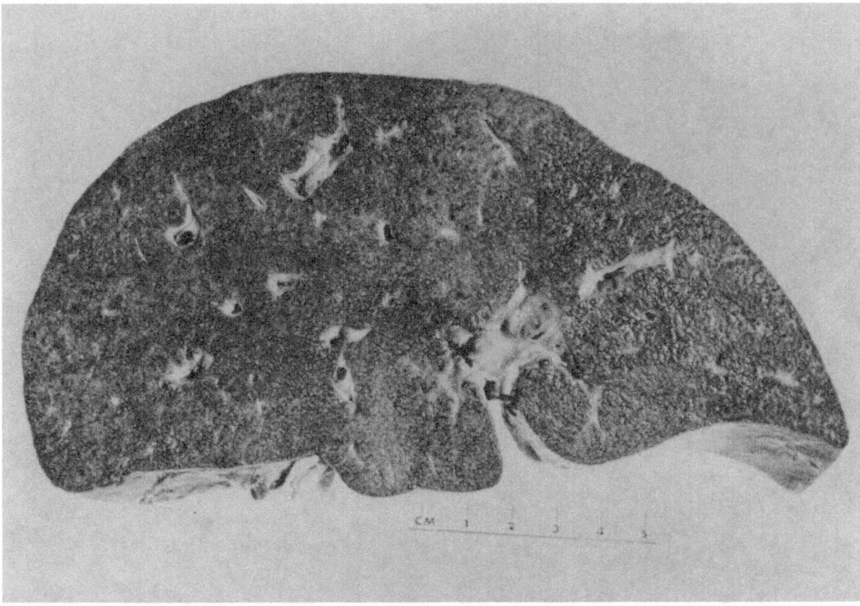

Fig. 7. Cirrhotic liver, from a patient with generalized histiocytosis X who died at age 26 months. This patient presented with jaundice.

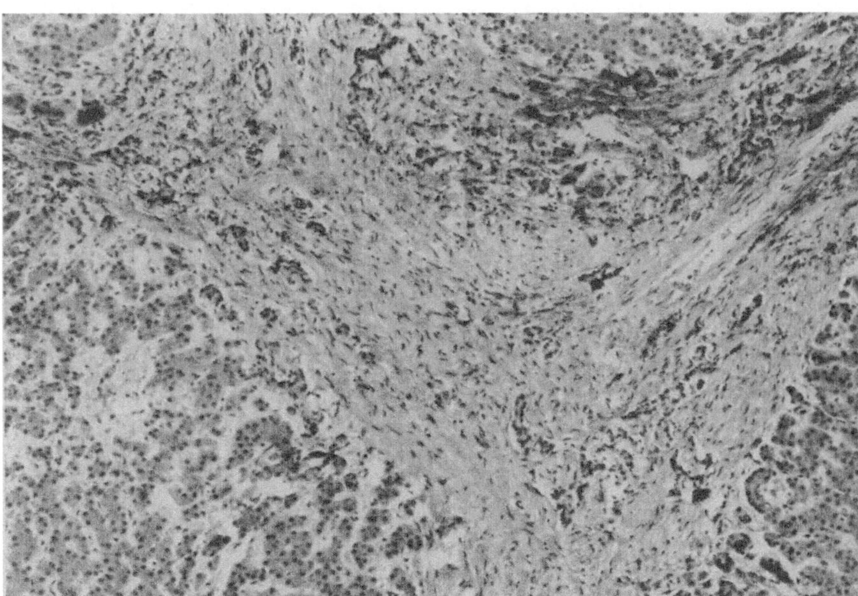

Fig. 8. Histological appearance of the liver shown in Fig. 7, with biliary cirrhosis. Some histiocytes are present in the scar tissue, but this infiltrate is not as heavy as seen in many cases. (x115)

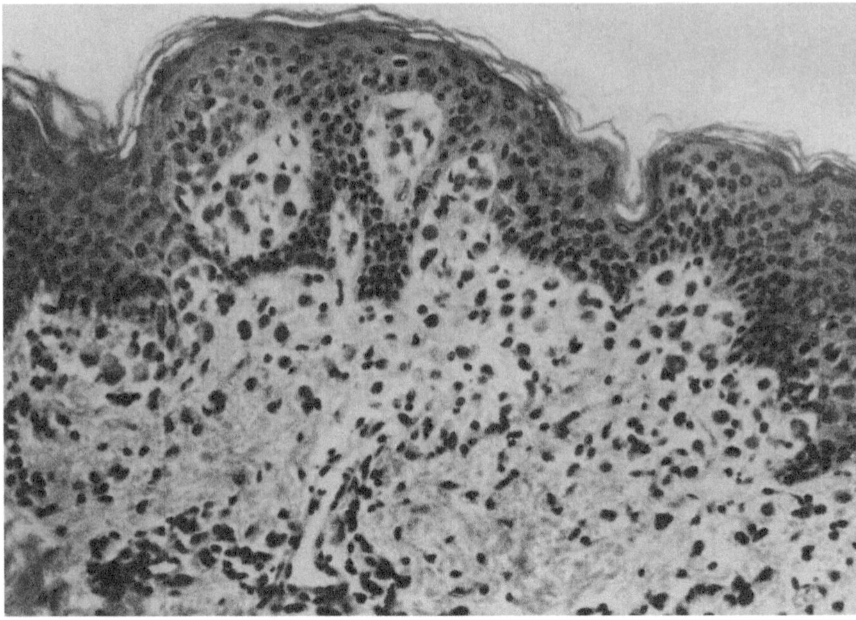

Fig. 9. Infiltrate of non-foamy histiocytes in the papillary dermis of the skin. This section shows no extension into the epidermis. (x290)

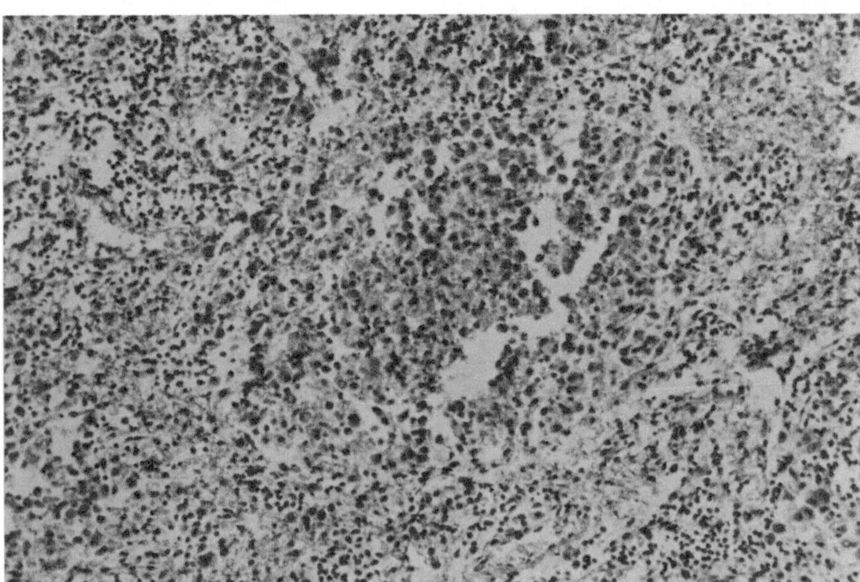

Fig. 10. Centrally necrotic infiltrate of histiocytes in the spleen of a rapidly fatal case of histiocytosis X. (x290)

Thymus

In the rapidly progressive cases, the thymus gland tended to be heavily and consistently involved with histiocytic infiltrates and was enlarged. In the slowly progressive cases, the thymus tended to be smaller than normal and had mild infiltrates of foam cells among the Hassal's corpuscles. In both groups, lymphoid tissue was greatly reduced as a consequence of stress.

Lung

Pulmonary infiltration with histiocytes was most prominent in the subpleural and peribronchial regions. Interstitial and intra-alveolar infiltrates were evident in some patients. In one of the cases with rapidly progressive disease there were many air-filled spaces because of destruction of lung tissue. The spaces were lined by a thin layer of histiocytes, some of which were foamy, and some giant cells.

Some survivors had radiographic evidence of pulmonary infiltration which eventually resolved or became smaller. As biopsies were not made of these lesions, their nature is uncertain.

Other Organs

In isolated cases, histiocytes infiltrated the thyroid, parathyroid, endocardium, tonsil, fat and choroid plexus.

Many patients, survivors and non-survivors, had clinical evidence of otitis media.

DISCUSSION

Lichtenstein[1] introduced the term histiocytosis X in 1953 to refer to a spectrum of disease ranging from eosinophilic granuloma of bone through Hand-Schüller-Christian syndrome to Letterer-Siwe disease. "Histiocytosis" implies that the histiocyte is the basic cell in the lesions and "X" designates the still-unidentified etiological agent.

Wallgren[2] in 1940 introduced the concept that this represents a single disease of variable severity and extent and proposed that Hand-Schüller-Christian syndrome and Letterer-Siwe disease were related entities. Eosinophilic granuloma of bone was first described in 1940[3,4]. In 1942, Green and Farber[5] classified all three entities as part of a single spectrum of disease.

The etiology remains unknown; it may be infectious, neoplastic, or due to a hypersensitivity reaction[6].

The Hand-Schüller-Christian syndrome was considered to be metabolic, but now most authorities agree that none of the disorders of the histiocytosis X group are related to specific biochemical abnormalities. The intracellular lipid is probably the result of phagocytosis.

Ultrastructural cytoplasmic inclusions have been described in histiocytes from the lesions of histiocytosis X[7,8]. They are rod-like structures with vesicular terminal enlargements and a dense central filament. Cross striations of variable periodicity are evident and the structures are sometimes branched. Some have interpreted these inclusions as viral. These structures are not specific for histiocytosis X. They were described initially in the Langerhans' cells of the epidermis in a patient with vitiligo. They might possibly be a cytoplasmic product, or may be stored material. Their morphology suggests that they are not viruses or phagocytosed debris.

The present study suggests that histiocytosis X is a continuous spectrum of disease both clinically and pathologically, extending from solitary eosinophilic granuloma of bone through multiple eosinophilic granuloma, to involvement of the extraskeletal tissues, to diffuse disease. When limited to the skeletal system, histiocytosis X was not fatal in this series. Cheyne[9] described a solitary vertebral lesion that produced spinal-cord compression and death by pyelonephritis. When the disease is entirely extraskeletal and involves many organ systems extensively, the prognosis is grave. Occasionally, patients have only limited extraskeletal-tissue involvement, then the prognosis is favourable. One child in the present series, whose only involvement was in multiple lymph nodes, had a favourable response to radiotherapy and the lesions did not recur. Similar cases have been described in other series[9].

The intermediate group – those patients with lesions of both the skeletal system and extraskeletal tissues, sometimes develop fatal disease, particularly patients under one year of age.

Rarely, patients who present with solitary eosinophilic granuloma of bone will develop diffuse extraskeletal involvement and die. In this series, three patients who were three months, five months, and 27 months old at the time of onset follow this course. The oldest patient had suffered from a rash for three months before he was seen with complaints referable to the lytic bone lesion. The other two developed evidence of extraskeletal-tissue involvement within a few months.

In most patients with eosinophilic granuloma of bone, the prognosis is favourable. Infants are more likely to develop additional lesions and extra-skeletal involvement than older children and adults, but histiocytosis X is rarely fatal when it develops after the third year of life (Fig. 11). In the present series, only one patient who died was over three years of age when the disease appeared. In contrast, a high percentage of patients whose histiocytosis X presented in the first year of life, ultimately died of the disease.

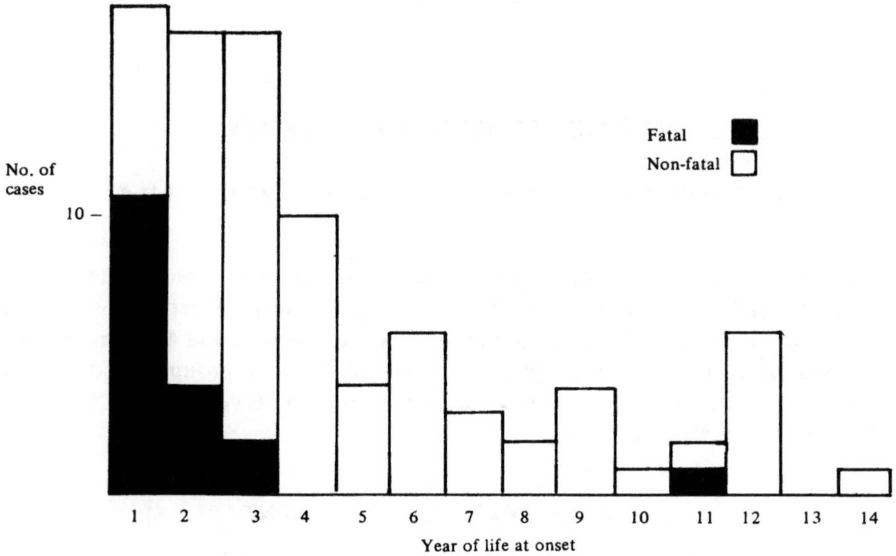

Fig. 11. Histiocytosis X (91 cases). age at onset.

REFERENCES

1 LICHTENSTEIN, L.. Histiocytosis X; integration of eosinophilic granuloma of bone, "Letterer-Siwe disease" and "Schüller-Christian disease" as related manifestations of single nosologic entity. *Arch Pathol,* **56**: 84, 1953.

2 WALLGREN, A.: Systemic reticuloendothelial granuloma: Nonlipoid reticuloendotheliosis and Schüller-Christian disease. *Am J Dis Child,* **60**: 471, 1940.

3 OTANI, S. and EHRLICH, J. C.. Solitary granuloma of bone simulating primary neoplasm. *Am J Pathol,* **16**: 479, 1940.

4 LICHTENSTEIN, L. and JAFFE, H. L.: Eosinophilic granuloma of bone, with report of case. *Am J Pathol,* **16**: 595, 1940.

5 GREEN, W. T. and FARBER, S.: "Eosinophilic or solitary granuloma" of bone. *J Bone Joint Surg,* **24**: 499, 1942.

6 LIEBERMAN, P. H., JONES, C. R. DARGEON, H. W. K. and BEGG, C. F.: A reappraisal of eosinophilic granuloma of bone, Hand-Schüller-Christian syndrome and Letterer-Siwe syndrome. *Medicine,* **48**: 375, 1969.

7 BASSET, F. and TURIAF, M. J.: Identification par la microscopie électronique de particules de nature probablement virale dans les liaisons granulomateuses d'une histiocytose "X" pulmonaire. *C R Acad Sci,* **261**: 3701, 1965.

8 De MAN, J. C. H.: Rod-like tubular structures in the cytoplasm of histiocytes in "histiocytosis X." *J Pathol Bacteriol,* **95**: 123, 1968.

9 CHEYNE, C.: Histiocytosis X. *J Bone Joint Surg, (Br),* **53**: 366, 1971.

HISTIOCYTOSIS X: MANAGEMENT

M. J. SONLEY, M.D., F.R.C.P.(C)* and F. GHAVIMI, M.D.**

One hundred and twenty-three patients with histiocytosis X were treated at the Hospital for Sick Children or the Princess Margaret Hospital between 1940 and 1970. Of these 123, 75 had involvement of a single system and 48 of more than one system at the time of diagnosis. The age of the total group ranged from 3 months to 50 years, but only three patients were over 16 years of age. The ratio of males to females was 1.9 to 1.

SINGLE SYSTEM INVOLVEMENT

In 75 patients only one system was involved at the time of diagnosis. The disease was confined to bone in 74, and one child had involvement of cervical, inguinal and axillary lymph glands.

The age range of these 75 was from eight months to 50 years with a median of five years. In contrast, the children who had involvement of several systems at the time of diagnosis, had a similar age range – from three months to 28 years – but the median age was only 22 months.

The presenting symptom was either pain or a lump over the involved site. Fifty-one children had a lesion in only one bone; nine had two bones involved, and 14 had lesions in several bones.

The skull, including orbits, was most commonly involved, with femurs, vertebrae and pelvis next in frequency (Table I).

Treatment

The patients were treated in a variety of ways. Table II shows the treatment given the 51 children who had only one lesion. One child had complete resection of a rib lesion; 27 children had their lesion curetted; 11 were treated with radiotherapy, and six had no treatment other than biopsy. When the patient had multiple lesions, the most accessible lesion was biopsied and then either curetted or radiated, or both. Lesions elsewhere were radiated if they were large, or in vital areas, such as the orbit or mastoid, or if there was a possibility the bone would fracture; otherwise they were observed and treated only if they progressed. No patient was treated with chemotherapy.

---

*Chief, Department of Pediatrics, The Princess Margaret Hospital, Toronto; Department of Hematology, The Hospital for Sick Children, Toronto; and Assistant Professor of Pediatrics, University of Toronto.

**Memorial Hospital for Cancer and Allied Diseases, New York, N.Y., U.S.A. (formerly of Department of Pediatrics, The Princess Margaret Hospital, Toronto.)

TABLE I
Single System
Site of Single Lesions

Skull or orbit	21
Femur	8
Vertebra	7
Pelvis	4
Tibia	3
Clavicle	2
Rib	2
Radius	1
Humerus	1
Sternum	1
Palate	1

TABLE II
Single System
Treatment

	1 Lesion	>1 Lesion
Resection	1	–
Curettage	27	5
XRT (radiation)	11	14
Curettage + XRT	6	5
Chemotherapy	–	–
Nil (5 had biopsy)	6	–
Total	51	24

The results of treatment were good irrespective of the method of treatment chosen (Table III). Local recurrence was infrequent. Surprisingly, there were more recurrences in children who were irradiated following curettage than in those who had curettage or radiotherapy alone, but the number so treated is too small to permit us to determine the significance of this observation.

TABLE III

Single Lesion
Local Recurrence

	No. of Lesions Treated	Local Recurrence
Resection	1	–
Curettage	27	1
XRT (radiation)	11	1
Curettage + XRT	6	3
Nil	6	1

Currently our choice of treatment depends on the location of the lesion. If it is in a site that can readily be curetted, such as in the skull, femur or tibia, and if the "quick" section confirms the diagnosis of histiocytosis X, the lesion is usually curetted under the same anesthetic. In bones not suitable for curettage, such as the mastoid, orbit, vertebrae or pelvis, biopsy is usually followed by radiotherapy. Multiple lesions are treated as described earlier; small lesions are observed and those in a vital area, or where a fracture appears imminent, are irradiated.

The dose of radiation necessary to control histiocytosis X is small (Table IV). Of the lesions treated with 600 rads or less, seven of 24 recurred, compared to only three of 29 lesions treated with 700-1000 rads, and three of 21 treated

TABLE IV

Histiocytosis X
Radiation Dose

Tumor Dose (rads)	No. of Lesions Treated	Local Recurrence No.	Local Recurrence Per cent
600 or less	24	7	(29)
7 – 800	9	1	(10)
9 – 1000	20	2	
11 – 1600	16	1	(14)
2 – 3000	5	2	

with 1100-3000 rads. There seems to be no advantage in increasing the dose of radiation above 1000 rads. We are currently giving a tumor dose of 800-1000 rads in four treatments.

Recurrences

The disease recurred locally in 12% of the 75 patients with single-system involvement. Distant recurrences were noted in 21% of patients who had only one bone involved at the time of diagnosis, compared to 58% if more than one lesion was present initially. Distant recurrences were usually in bone. Diabetes insipidus developed in four patients and one child developed an infiltrate in the lung. The time until the recurrence was detected varied from one to 87 months, with a median of 10 months.

Fifteen patients had only one recurrence, six had two separate episodes of recurrence, while three had three episodes and one had four.

As mentioned previously, new lesions were treated with radiotherapy according to the location and size of the lesion. None of the patients were given chemotherapy at any time during their course.

Prognosis

No deaths have been known to have occurred due to histiocytosis X in the 75 patients with single-system involvement, although one patient died seven years later of synovial sarcoma at a different site, and one patient was lost to follow-up after operation. Five patients were followed less than two years, 68 patients were followed at least two years – 34 of them for more than five years – and all were well and free of disease when last heard from.

MULTIPLE SYSTEM DISEASE

Forty-eight patients had more than one system involved at the time of diagnosis. We attempted to divide the patients into those with acute disseminated disease and those with chronic disseminated disease, but in many the course was so variable that it was impossible to decide, at the time of presentation, whether they were going to run an acute or chronic course. Some patients started slowly with otitis media and a rash occurring intermittently over several months, and then developed an acute fulminating illness and died. Others started with acute fulminating disease and then settled down to a prolonged course with involvement of various bones or organs over a period of months or years – some ultimately dying of their disease while in others it eventually regressed completely.

The most common presenting symptoms were a rash, otitis media or externa, fever and ulcers in mucous membranes (Table V). At the time of diagnosis two-thirds of the patients had a rash and approximately one-half had hepatomegaly and enlarged nodes (Table VI). To indicate the extent of disease at diagnosis, we assigned one point to the patient for each physical finding or laboratory value listed in Table VI. If all of the findings were present, the child could have a maximum score of 12.

TABLE V

Multi System Presenting Symptoms – 48 Patients

Rash	24
Otitis	14
Fever	14
Ulcer – gums 5 – anus 4 – vulva 1	10
Mass	8
Polyuria + polydipsia	5
Resp. symptoms	4
Nodes	4
Proptosis	3
Pain	2
Upper respiratory infection	2
Loose teeth	2
Stiff neck	1
Vertigo	1

TABLE VI

Multi System Signs at Diagnosis – 48 Patients

Rash	31
Liver	26
Nodes	24
Spleen	19
Otitis	18
Ulcer – gums 8 – anus 4 – vulva 1	13
Diabetes insipidus	9
Bone lesions (x-ray)	34
Hgb <10	20
Lung infiltrate (x-ray)	14
Platelets <100.000	11
Bone marrow positive for tumor cells (20 aspirations)	2

Treatment

The treatment varied tremendously. These patients presented over a period of 30 years and some were diagnosed only at autopsy or on routine review of tissue sections several years after the illness began. During this period effective chemotherapeutic agents were gradually discovered and the ancillary care also improved – with better antibiotics, platelet transfusions, etc. Ten patients had no specific treatment and two of them survived (Table VII). Of the 16 patients who had only radiotherapy throughout their course, 14 survived. None of the five patients who received only chemotherapy survived, whereas 12 of 17 who had a combination of chemotherapy and radiotherapy were alive five years later. Comparison of the extent-of-disease scores reveals that those patients who had only chemotherapy had the most severe involvement, while those who had radiotherapy alone had the least extensive disease. Optimal treatment is probably chemotherapy with radiation to resistant lesions or to lesions where a rapid response is important, e.g., an impending fracture, exophthalmos, mastoid destruction.

TABLE VII

Multi System
Histiocytosis X

Treatment	No. of Pts.	Alive	Involvement Score	
			Range	Median
None	10	2	2 – 8	4
XRT (radiation)	16	14	2 – 8	3
Chemotherapy	5	–	5 – 9	7
XRT + Chemotherapy	17	12	2 – 10	6

Chemotherapy was usually given as a single drug (Table VIII). Most frequently prednisone was used first and produced temporary complete regression of disease in three of the 15 patients in whom the response could be assessed, and some improvement in two-thirds of the patients. Methotrexate, vincoleukoblastine, cyclophosphamide and vincristine have each produced complete or partial regression in one-third to one-half of the patients where the response could be assessed. More recently two drugs have been given simultaneously, for example, deltacortisone (prednisone) and vinblastine sulfate (Velbe) with a 50% remission rate. Because the disease tends to recur if the drug is discontinued immediately after a response is noted, currently we are keeping the children on chemotherapy for three to six months after all signs of active disease have disappeared.

TABLE VIII

Multi System
Histiocytosis X – Chemotherapy

	No. of Pts.	CR	PR	Total CR + PR
Prednisone	15	3	7	10/15
Methotrexate	9	2	3	5/9
Vincoleukoblastine	6	1	1	2/6
Cyclophosphamide	2	1	–	1/2
Vincristine	2	–	1	1/2

Nineteen patients developed diabetes insipidus, which was present at diagnosis in 10 and was diagnosed later in nine. All had skull x-rays but only one patient had a lesion in the area of sella turçica. Since pathologic changes have been found infrequently in the pituitary at autopsy, it is difficult to decide whether patients who develop diabetes insipidus should have their pituitaries radiated (Table IX). Eleven of our patients had pituitary irradiation while eight did not. Subsequently, two children in each group had a decrease in symptoms. One patient who did not have radiotherapy and two who were irradiated never developed symptoms severe enough to require pitressin. However, in the remainder, the diabetes insipidus continued unchanged irrespective of whether they were irradiated or not. No patients developed signs of progressive disease such as involvement of the anterior pituitary. The development of diabetes insipidus is not a bad prognostic sign – only three of these patients died and these deaths occurred 20 months, 7 years, and 11 years after the diagnosis of histiocytosis X. An evaluation of our patients does not reveal whether a child who develops diabetes insipidus should have irradiation to his pituitary.

TABLE IX

Diabetes Insipidus

19 Patients

4 Single System / 15 Multi - System

Alive – 16

Onset	At diagnosis – 10	(up to 14 yrs. before)
	After diagnosis – 9	(11 – 72 months later) Median – 26
Treatment	XRT to pituitary – 11	
	None – 8	

Result		No Treatment	XRT
	Still on pitressin	5 (1 died)	7 (2 died)
	Pitressin discontinued	2	2
	Never on pitressin	1	2
	Total	8	11

Dead 3 (after 20 mo., 7 and 11 yr.)

Survival

The prognosis depends on the age of the patient and the extent of the disease at diagnosis. The patients' "extent-of-disease" scores ranged from 2 to 10 at the time of diagnosis (Table X). Ninety per cent of those who had a score of 2 or 3 were alive and well five years after the diagnosis and even when the score was 6 to 10, 25 to 30% survived five years. These figures are lower than one should expect with current therapy because they were treated by various modes; and some patients, treated many years ago, received no therapy. The figures demonstrate, however, that even with extensive disease at diagnosis the prognosis is certainly not hopeless.

The age at diagnosis was also important in the prognosis. Eleven of the 24 children under two years survived five years, compared to 13 of the 17 children over two years of age. The survival rate for the whole group was 58% (Table XI).

Two patients died more than five years after diagnosis. One boy died of his disease in 1958, 10 years after diagnosis, and another died, in 1968, of exudative enteropathy due to methotrexate toxicity, seven years after diagnosis.

The five-year survival rate has improved with each decade since the disease was recognized and, since 1960, 16 of the 18 patients followed for two years and 11 of the 12 patients followed for five years are alive (Fig. 1). This improvement is likely due to many factors. The diagnosis is being made earlier because of a higher index of suspicion among pediatricians and because of the ease of needle biopsy of the skin. Improvement in the supportive care, the development of new and better chemotherapeutic agents, and the more optimistic and aggressive approach to the treatment have all contributed to the improvement in prognosis.

TABLE X

Survival According to Score at Diagnosis

Score	2	3	4	5	6	7	8	9	10
No. of Patients	10	8	7	5	6	3	4	2	3
Alive	9	7	4	2	2	1	1	1	1

TABLE XI

Multi System
Histiocytosis X
5-Year Survival (According to Age at Diagnosis)

Age Years	Total Cases	Evaluable	Alive at 5 Yrs.	Per cent Survival
<1	12	10	4	46
1	15	14	7	
2	7	7	6	76
3 or 4	8	7	5	
5+	6	3	2	
Total	48*	41	24	58

*5 not followed 5 yrs.
2 lost to follow-up.

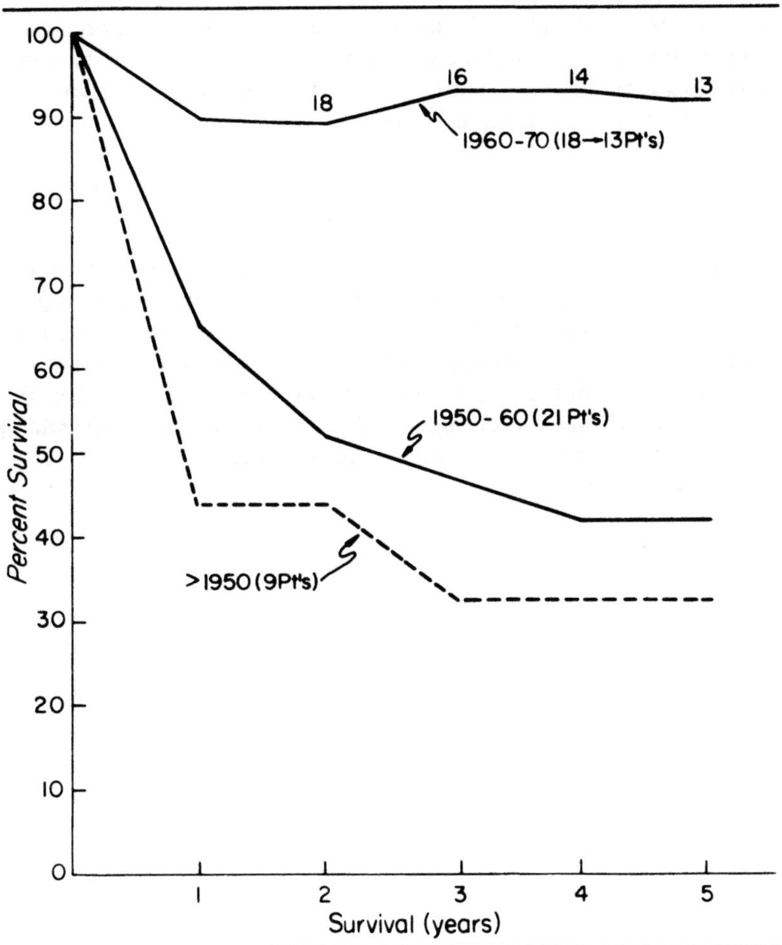

Fig. 1. Multiple system – histiocytosis X.

CONCLUSION

Histiocytosis X, when confined to bone at the time of diagnosis, is a self-limited benign disease. Because at least 20% of patients with this disease will develop distant lesions, they should be followed for several years after diagnosis. However, the ultimate result is excellent and treatment should not be too aggressive.

Generalized histiocytosis X involving multiple systems is more severe. The prognosis is not as good in children under two years of age, or in those with extensive disease at diagnosis, but as the treatment has become more aggressive and optimistic the prognosis has improved.

ADDENDUM

Surprisingly, of the five patients with multiple-system disease diagnosed since November 1970, four have done extremely poorly, two infants who presented with severe cirrhosis which was already sufficient to lead to their demise, died of concurrent infections. A third, aged 12 months at diagnosis, died of infection superimposed on pulmonary infiltration with histiocytosis X, and a fourth child, diagnosed at four months of age, died eight months later of widespread histiocytosis X despite progressively more intensive radiotherapy and chemotherapy.

RADIOTHERAPY OF NASOPHARYNGEAL ANGIOFIBROMA

P. J. FITZPATRICK, M.B., F.F.R., F.R.C.P.(C)*
and W. D. RIDER, M.B., F.F.R., F.R.C.P.(C)**

Review of the literature on the rare nasopharyngeal angiofibroma reveals a number of inconsistencies in the tumor's spectrum, its behaviour and its response to treatment[1-5]. Accordingly, we studied patients with this lesion seen at the Princess Margaret Hospital, Toronto, in order to draw conclusions about these inconsistencies and reported our findings in 1967 and 1970[6,7]. The series is now larger and consists of 39 patients. The follow-up period has also increased and we have gained further experience with the radiological and endocrine investigation in these patients. Although we have reported previously on the juvenile angiofibroma of the nasopharynx, our further experience has done much to crystallize our thinking about tumor behaviour and its management.

MATERIALS AND METHODS

Between 1946 and 1971, 39 patients were seen with nasopharyngeal angiofibroma – 36 were male and three female (Table I). The median age for males was 14 years, 8 months, and ranged from nine to 28 years. The females were 14, 19 and 36 years old. Most patients had severe symptoms for two to 48 months before diagnosis (Table II). Most had epistaxis and nasal obstruction, and facial deformity from swelling of the cheek and invasion of the orbit. Ten patients required transfusion for uncontrolled bleeding, which was either spontaneous or aggravated by surgical intervention.

GENERAL OBSERVATIONS

Pathology

The tumor is usually nodular and dark red with evidence of recent hemorrhage. There is no true capsule but compression of the normal tissues produces a pseudocapsule. Tissue was available for study in all cases and, histologically, the tumor consists of vascular connective tissue which becomes more fibrous with age. The blood vessels, which are dilated, have incomplete muscle coats and may only have a single endothelial layer of cells.

---

*Princess Margaret Hospital, Toronto; and Assistant Professor of Therapeutic Radiology, University of Toronto.

**Princess Margaret Hospital, Toronto; and Associate Professor of Therapeutic Radiology, University of Toronto.

TABLE I

Juvenile Nasopharynx Angiofibroma*

1946 - 1971

	Age	Duration Of Symptoms
Male 36*	14 yrs. 8 mos. median 9 - 28 range	1 yr. median 2 mos. - 4 yrs. range
Female 3	14, 19, 36 yrs.	

** 1 patient treated with radium 1919 → 40 years later developed ca. nasopharynx

1 patient died at angiography untreated

*All patients seen at Princess Margaret Hospital 1946-1971.

**Patient treated elsewhere in 1919 received a minimum dose of 60,000 rads.

TABLE II

Nasopharyngeal Angiofibroma

PRESENTING SYMPTOMS

38 PATIENTS

	No. Of Patients		No. Of Patients
Epistaxis	31	Swelling of Cheek	9
Nasal Obstruction		Proptosis	4
Unilateral	28	Impaired Vision	1
Bilateral	9	Impaired Hearing	3
Mouth Breathing	1	Headache	4
Nasal Voice	4		
Nasal Discharge	5		

Endocrine Assessment

Special studies were done in 17 males and two females to determine maturation, genetic and endocrine status. Because many patients were mouth breathers with a nasal voice, and some swelling of the eyelids, they gave the appearance of having a low I.Q. However, this was not substantiated, although four children were backward at school and one exhibited psychopathic behaviour. The results of the clinical investigations and laboratory tests (Tables III-V) were all within the normal range.

TABLE III

Angiofibroma Assessment*

Age	Bone Age
Weight	Hair Distribution
Height	Testicle Size
Crown to Pubis	Penile Length
Pubis to Heel	Buccal Smear (chromosomes)
Span	
Parents }	Height
Siblings }	Age

*Factors measured in the clinical assessment for endocrine status. All were normal.

TABLE IV

Nasopharyngeal Angiofibroma*

HISTORY

Age of Onset:

Hair
- Axillary
- Pubic
- Facial
- Temporal (Regression)

1st Erection

1st Nocturnal Emission (♀ 1st period)

Change in Voice

1st Sign Acne

*These specific facts were recorded in the endocrine assessment. All were normal.

TABLE V

Nasopharyngeal Angiofibroma*

Urinary Excretion

FSH

Estrogen

17 - KS

17 - OHCS

—

Plasma - Serum

Cortisol 8:30 am.
4:40 pm.

Testosterone

Thryoxine

—

24 hr. Thryoidal ^{131}I uptake

T3 uptake

*Pituitary activity was assessed by these laboratory tests. All were within normal limits.

Radiology

Radiographs of the skull were taken in all patients and included posteroanterior, lateral, base and soft-tissue lateral views. These films demonstrate the tumor but do not reveal its total extent or whether it has damaged bone. Coronal polytomography reveals both tumor extension and bone damage that may not be suspected on clinical examination or the study of routine films. Carotid arteriography clearly demonstrates the vessels of the tumor but rarely delineates the spread into the air sinuses or cranium. Twenty-eight patients were studied by arteriography. The main blood supply is from the internal maxillary artery, which is often grossly enlarged, although other vessels, notably the opthalmic artery, may contribute to the blood supply. Most tumors received their blood from one carotid system only but, in three patients, there was a contribution from both sides. The diagnostic radiology required to demonstrate a tumor is shown in Figs. 1-3.

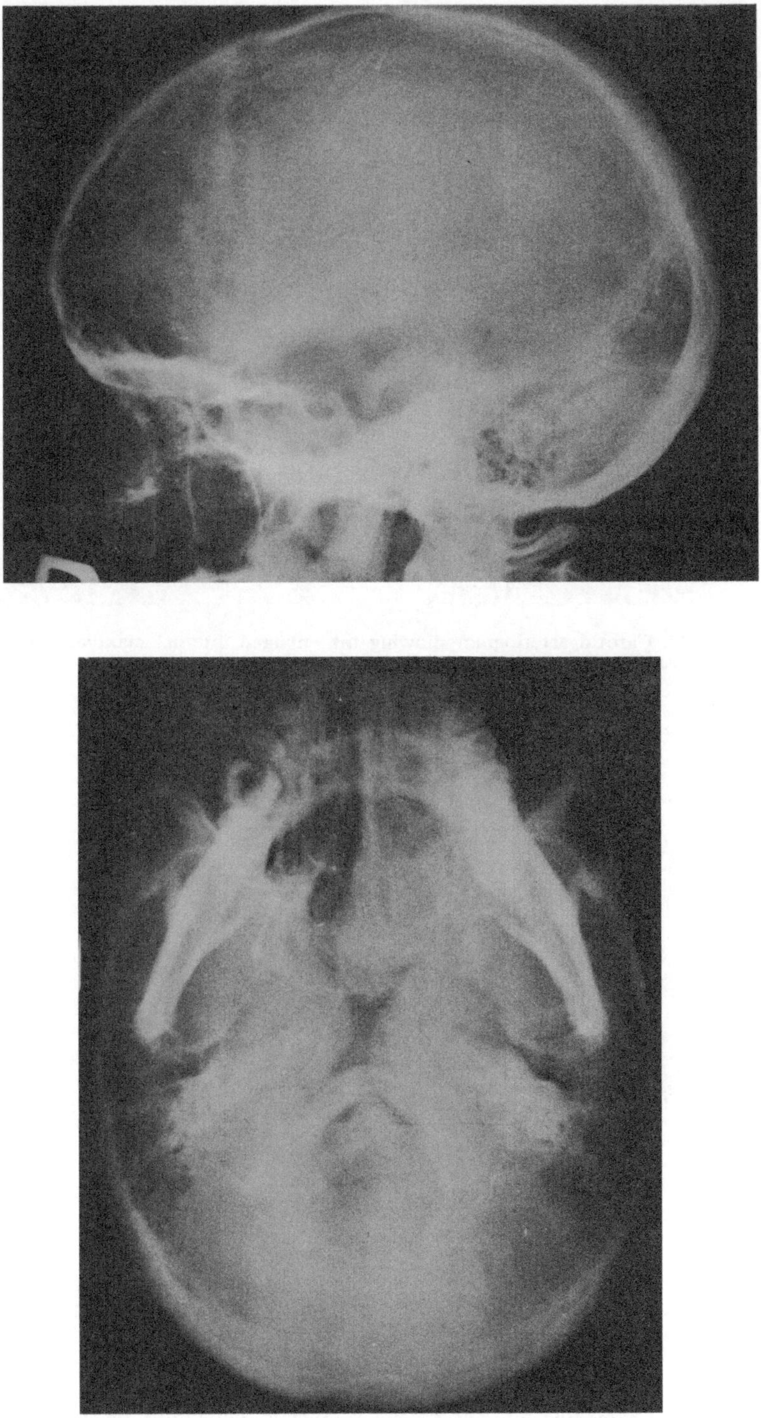

Fig. 1. Case 37. Radiographs of lateral and base of skull. Note large soft-tissue mass in nasopharynx, left side of nose and hazy appearance of sphenoid air sinus.

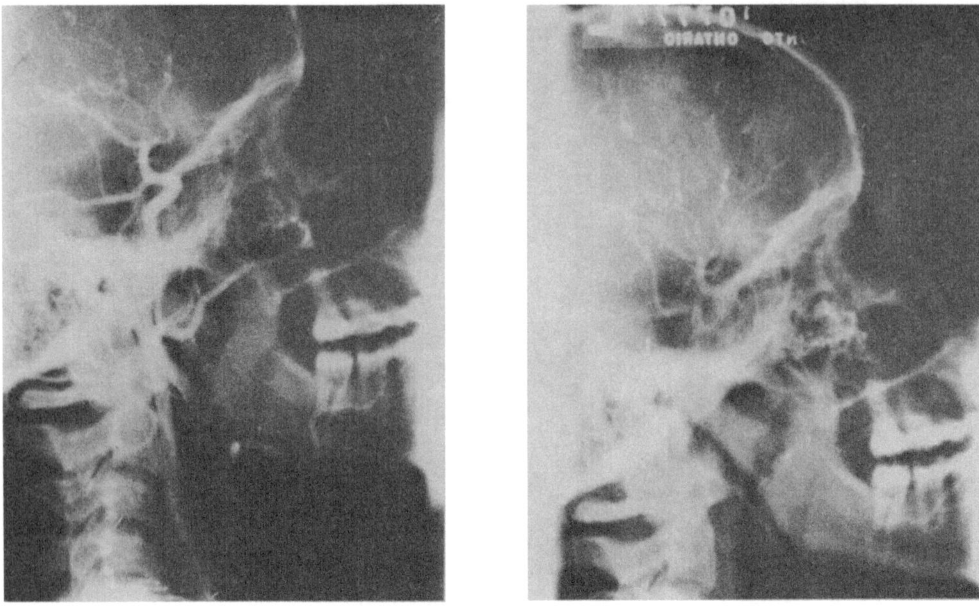

Fig. 2. Case 37. Carotid arteriogram showing the enlarged internal maxillary artery and extensive vascular supply to tumor in the nasopharynx.

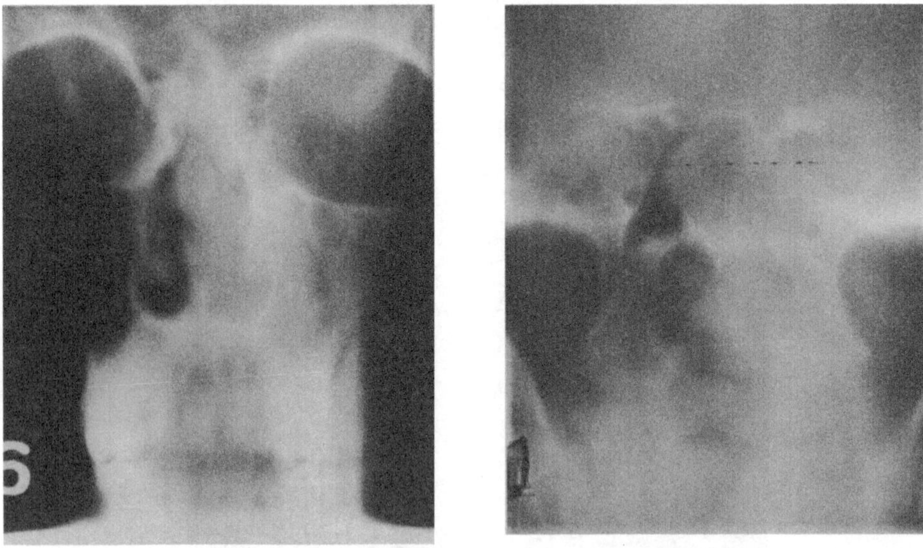

Fig. 3. Case 37. The serial coronal tomograms clearly show the large tumor mass eroding bone and extending into the sphenoid, ethmoid and antrum on the left side. We found this the most useful investigation.

Recent advances in diagnostic radiology have made it clear that this tumor destroys bone at the base of the skull much more commonly than previously considered (Table VI). In the total series, 30 of 38 patients had bone destruction and this figure may have been higher had all patients had tomography. Among the last 26 patients, only two did not have bone erosion or tumor spread into one of the accessory air sinuses. More than one bone was eroded in 22 patients; the tumor had also spread into the orbit or cranium in nine patients.

Treatment

Initially, 18 of 37 patients were treated surgically before being referred to Princess Margaret Hospital (Table VII). These 18 had submitted to 42 attempts at resection without tumor control and their symptoms were severe enough to warrant referral to our hospital. Nineteen patients had received no previous treatment. Subsequently these 37 were treated by irradiation to a dose of 3000 to 3500 rads in 14 to 16 fractions over a three-week period. Thirty-three patients were irradiated with a supervoltage unit (Table VIII). Following irradiation, all had early symptomatic relief, but often many months passed before objective tumor regression became apparent. Six patients had persistent or recurrent tumor which required further intervention (Table IX). In two patients, the tumor was too extensive to consider operation and they received a second course of radiotherapy with a good result. Four patients with recurrent tumor underwent resection; in two, this failed to control the tumor and they were re-irradiated with tumor control. The initial side effects of radiation were minimal and disappeared soon after its completion. No serious complications of treatment were recorded.

We decided to observe rather than treat two patients with minimal symptoms but, within a few months, the tumors grew rapidly and irradiation had to be given. Three patients were treated with androgens without any detectable improvement.

TABLE VI

Angiofibroma Bone Involvement*

30/38	Patients	-	Bone Erosion	
24/26	Patients	-	Tomography	Bone Erosion
22	Patients	-	Multiple Bones Involved	
			Sphenoid	25
			Antrum	19
			Ethmoids	17
			Orbit	5
			Cranium	4

*Tumor infiltration to the air sinuses was common and in many patients only demonstrated by tomography.

TABLE VII

Summary of Treatment
37 Patients with Nasopharyngeal Angiofibroma

RESULTS

23/37 Patients followed > 5 yrs.

1st Treatment	No.		Control*
Surgery (42 operations)	19	Radiation →	15/19
Radiation	18		16/18

7 Patients followed < 2yrs. appear controlled
7 Patients lost to follow up at 2 yrs.

*After irradiation only six patients required further treatment.

TABLE VIII

Summary of Radiotherapy of Nasopharyngeal Angiofibroma

TREATMENT

	No.	Technique		No.
Radiation	37			
^{60}Co.	31		Parallel Pair	21
400 KV	3	Fields	Wedge	6
270 KV	1		Three	10
22 MeV electrons	1			
22 MeV X-ray	1			

Tumour Dose 3000 rds - 15 Rx - 3/52

TABLE IX

Further Treatment of Patients with Symptomatic Tumors after Irradiation

	RESULTS			
Recurrence after Radiation	Treatment	Control	Treatment	Control*
6	Surgery 4	2/4	Radiation	2/2
	Radiation 2	2/2		

*Radiation was required in four of the six for complete control.

DISCUSSION

Because of the tendency to severe hemorrhage, biopsy must be obtained in the operating room under anesthetic with full surgical and transfusion facilities available.

One patient died during arteriography – probably due to an anesthetic idiosyncrasy. Autopsy revealed an enormous, red, lobulated, vascular tumor about 6.0 cm. in diameter, which filled the nasopharynx and destroyed the sphenoid sinus. The tumor also filled the pituitary fossa and the recesses of the wings of the sphenoid. This tragic experience and the revelations of more sophisticated radiology have convinced us that these tumors are invariably much larger than they appear at first sight and that most of our failures can be attributed to a "geographic miss", the situation when some of the tumor is omitted from the irradiated volume.

The patients managed early in this series were treated with a pair of simple parallel radiation fields. In retrospect, the good results previously reported may have been due to luck, because tomography was not done in most of them and the radiation fields were comparatively small. In 1964 we investigated two patients who did not respond to radiotherapy and found that the treatment fields did not encompass the total tumor and, in particular, omitted most of the sphenoidal sinus. Because of the widespread ramifications of the tumor and the importance of total coverage, treatment must be planned individually, giving full protection to the radiovulnerable structures such as the anterior chamber of the eye and the cervical cord. The radiotherapy techniques used for different situations are shown in Figs. 4-8. Homogenous radiation at the points of interest calls for elegant techniques including the use of wedges and multiple fields with casts and compensators. Fig. 8 shows the treatment plan for the second course of irradiation given to Case 24. The first course of irradiation with a pair of simple parallel cobalt-60 fields was given after an attempt at resection had failed. The patient had some immediate symptomatic relief but, in the next year, the tumor mass increased, eroded the sphenoid and orbit and produced complete nasal obstruction, epistaxis and proptosis. Accordingly, a technique was devised to limit radiation to the normal structures while covering the new tumor extensions. After the second course of irradiation, there was symptomatic improvement but it was not complete for nearly one year (Fig. 9a and 9b).

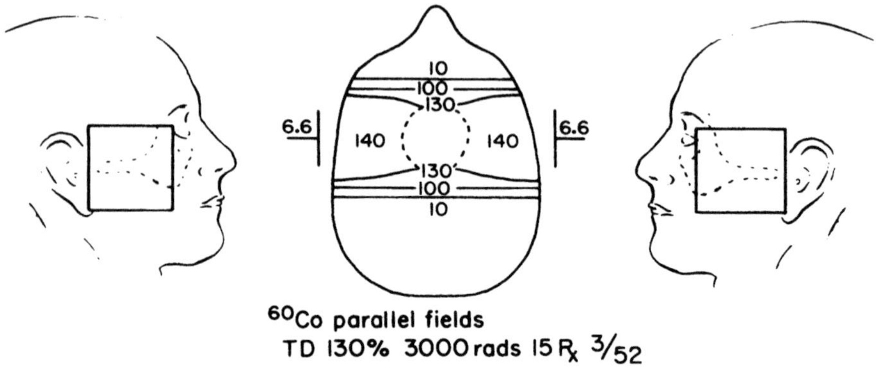

Fig. 4. The simplest radiation technique for the average tumor.

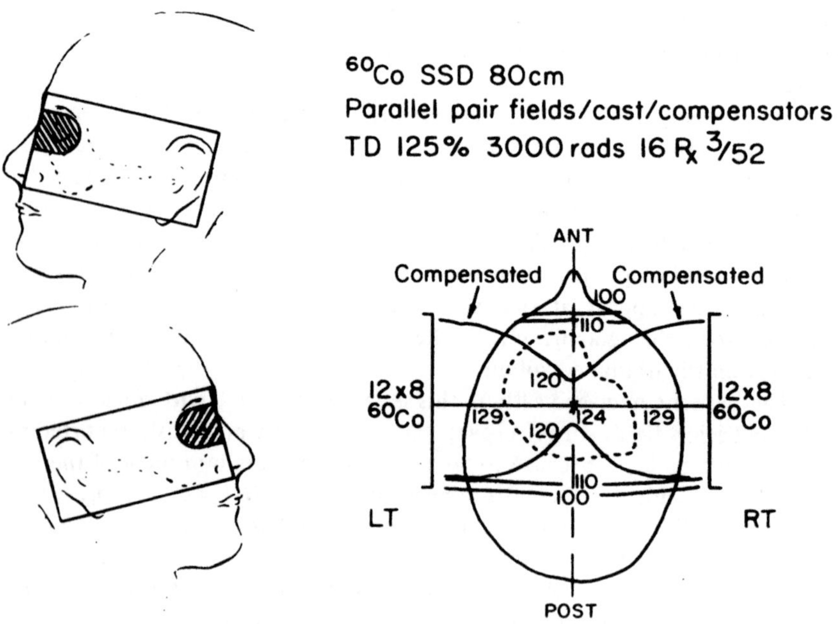

Fig. 5. A more sophisticated radiotherapy technique for patients with large tumors extending into the nose.

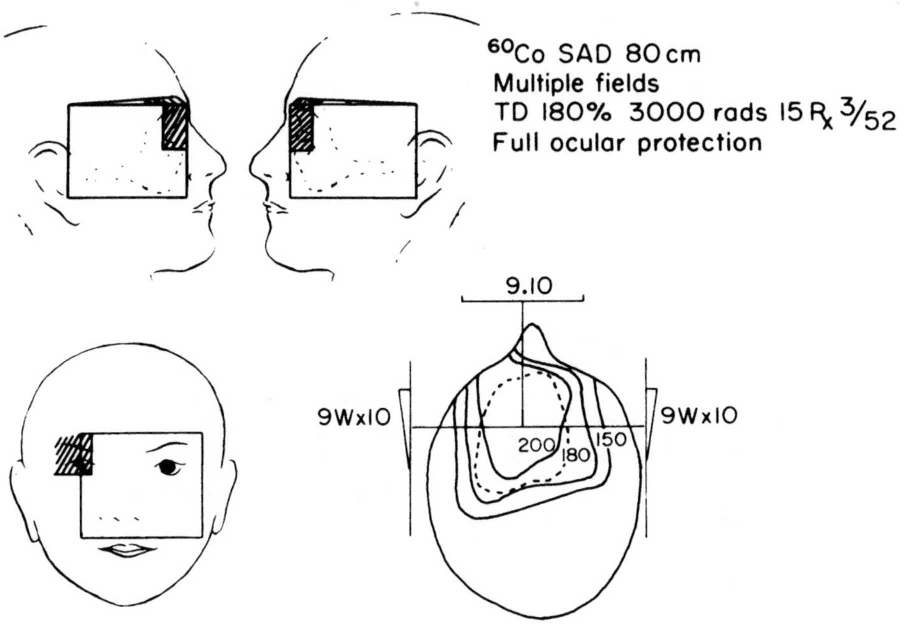

Fig. 6. A three-field radiotherapy technique used for large tumors that have infiltrated to one side.

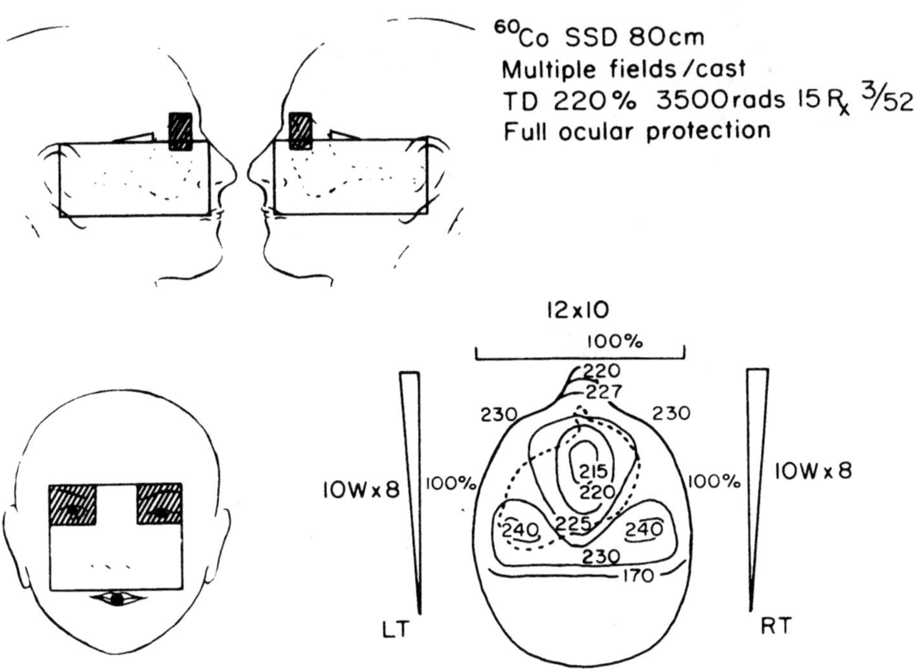

Fig. 7. A three-field radiotherapy technique used for massive tumors that have infiltrated widely in all directions.

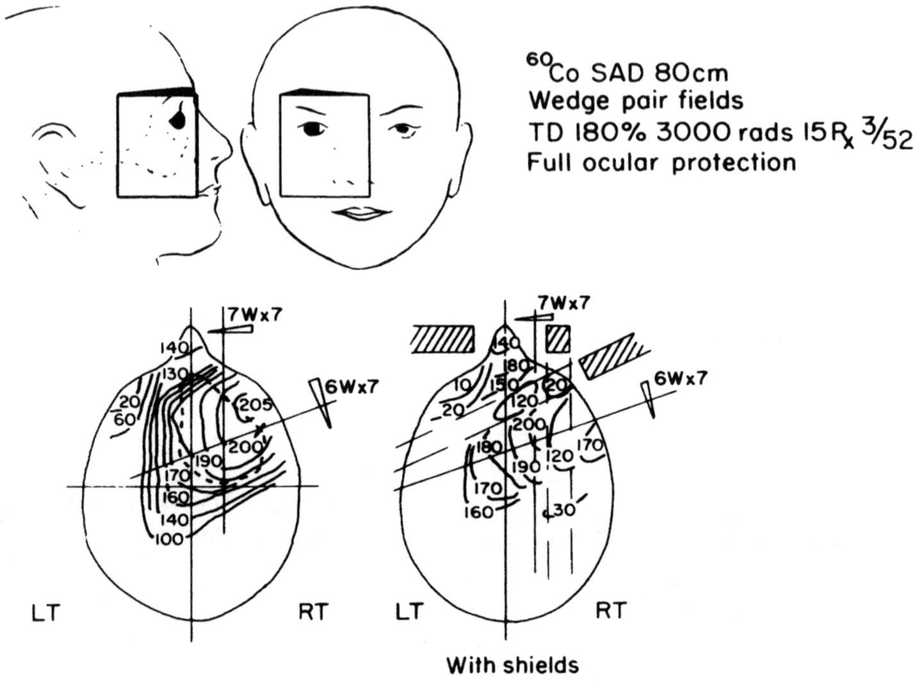

Fig. 8. A wedge pair radiotherapy technique used to treat Case 24. This patient was treated by surgery, radiotherapy, two further operations and a second course of radiotherapy before his tumor was controlled.

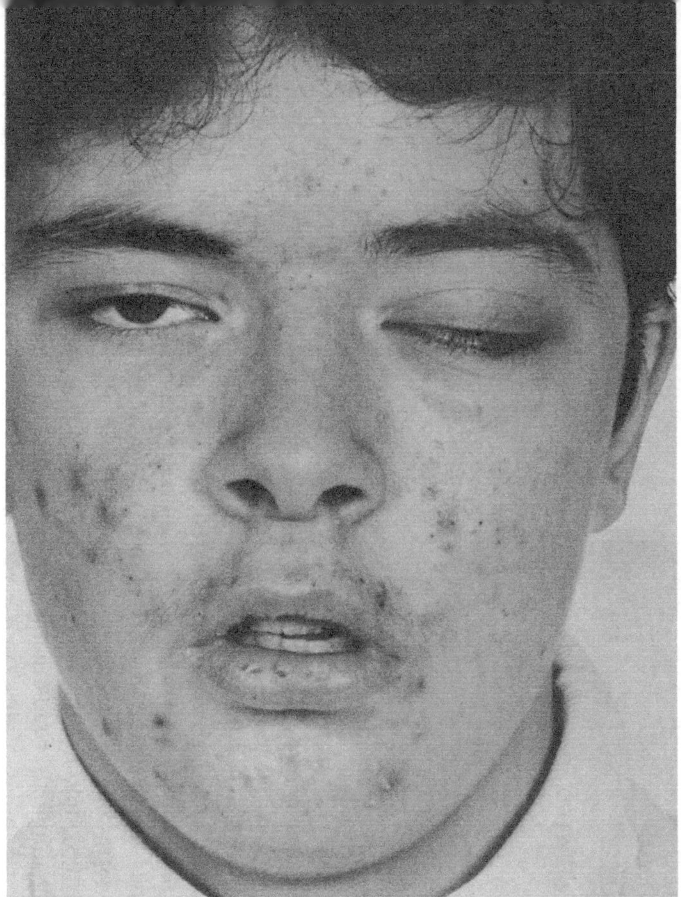

Fig. 9a. Case 24. Recurrence with complete nasal obstruction and proptosis after three operations and a course of radiotherapy. The second course of irradiation 18 months later produced immediate symptomatic relief.

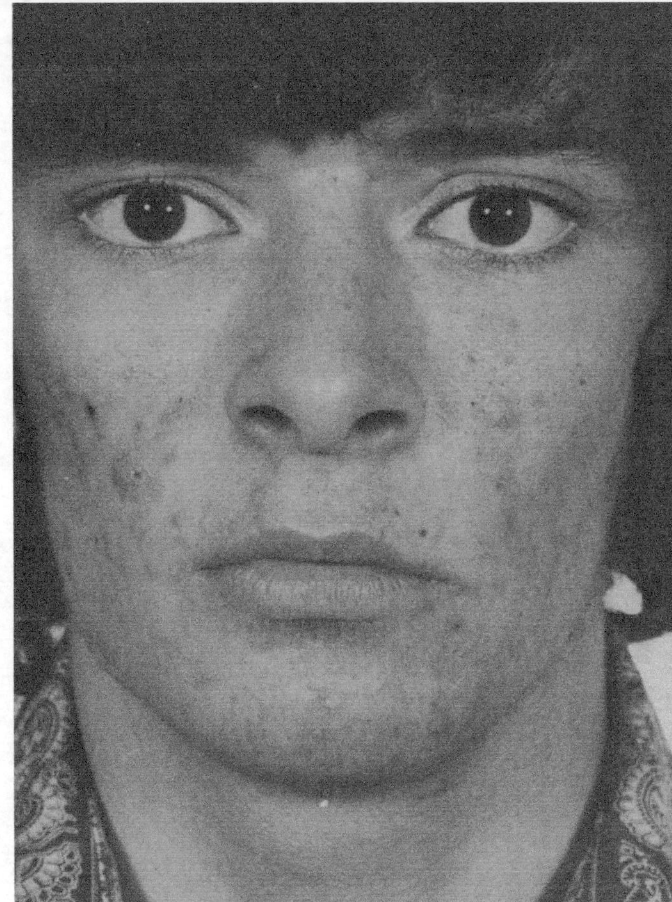

Fig. 9b. Case 24. Four years after first operation and two years after second course of radiotherapy.

Regression of tumor following irradiation is clearly demonstrated by Case 31 (Figs. 10a and 10b). This patient had the most extensive tumor that we have seen and had massive intracranial extension that necessitated a craniotomy because of decreasing vision. However, the tumor was too extensive for any surgical procedure and radiotherapy was commenced immediately. At the end of treatment, the patient, who was nearly blind on admission, could read large letters and distinguish figures on a cornflakes box. Since then, the left eye has remained blind with optic atrophy but the right eye has normal vision of 20/20.

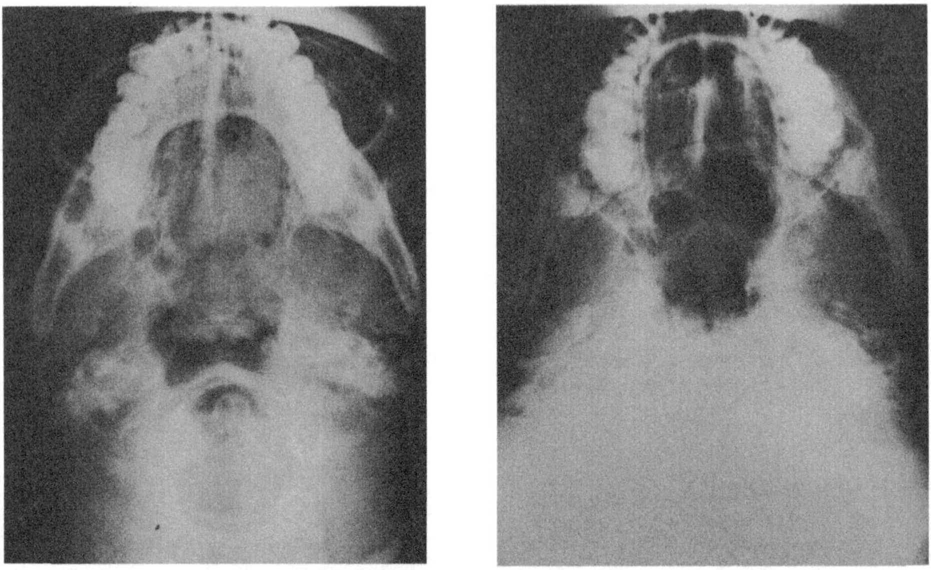

Figs. 10a & 10b. Case 31. Radiographs of the base of the skull showing a large angiofibroma (a) before and (b) one year after Co^{60} irradiation with a dose of 3000 rads in three weeks. The patient had massive intra-cranial extension by tumor and was almost blind at commencement of radiotherapy. His right eye recovered to 20/20 vision but his left eye remained blind with optic atrophy.

Our philosophy of non-interference following radiotherapy was confirmed after Case 13 was treated in 1964. This patient lived more than 1000 miles away on an island in the St. Lawrence estuary where specialist medical surveillance was not available. On completion of irradiation, although the tumor had shown some regression, the patient still had symptoms: because of the distance involved, he was given a six-month return appointment. At that time, the tumor was about one-half its original size and his symptoms had nearly disappeared. We decided to review the situation after a further six months; at this time the tumor had regressed to a residual nubbin on the roof of the nasopharynx and the patient symptom free. Since that time, our policy has been to avoid all tumor intervention after radiotherapy although it is sometimes difficult to persuade surgeons to desist when symptomatic patients have a mass in the nasopharynx.

The radiographs of Case 20 (Figs. 11-12) demonstrate this point. This patient had a large tumor in the nasopharynx extending into the left side of the nose which regressed in a satisfactory manner following irradiation. However, serial radiographs taken over the next two years showed a residual nubbin of tumor in the region of the left posterior choana, which was probably its site of origin. This residuum does not require treatment and this picture has been seen in several patients. We do not believe that this is evidence of spontaneous tumor regression because all of our patients were irradiated. We attempted to observe two patients without treatment but increasing symptoms required treatment. Every patient had some symptomatic improvement on the completion of radiotherapy. Some had a latent period of months before relief of symptoms was complete. Years after treatment, meticulous examination and tomographic radiology will detect a residual mass in some patients.

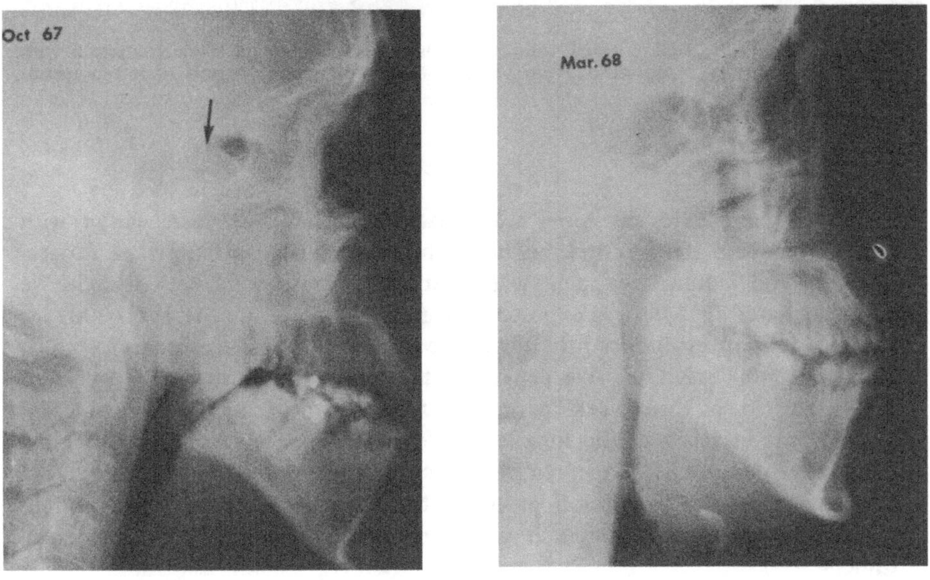

Fig. 11. Case 20. Lateral skull radiographs before and six months after irradiation. Note tumor regression.

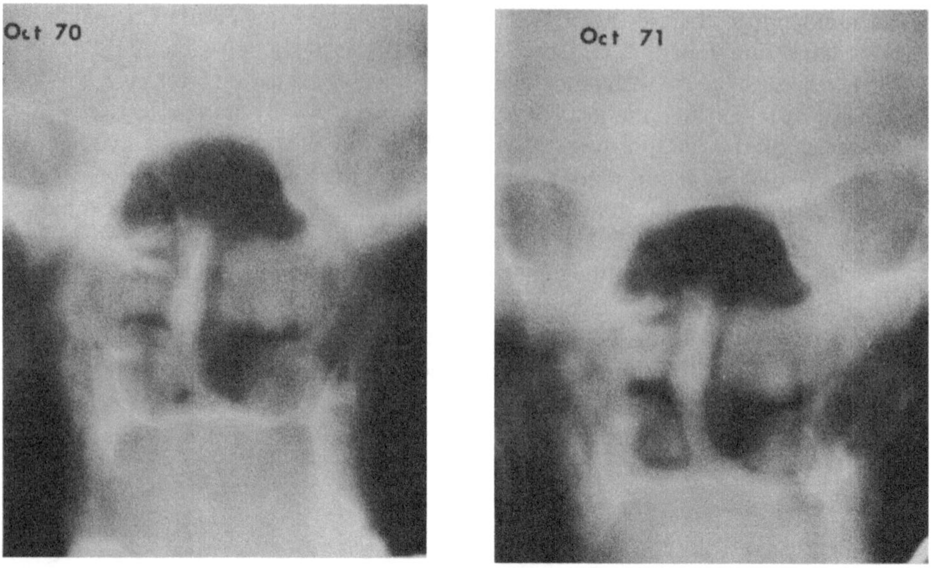

Fig. 12. Case 20. Serial coronal tomograms three and four years after irradiation with patient asymptomatic. Note residual tumor nubbin in region of left posterior choana.

One patient in the series was treated elsewhere 40 years earlier with radium plaques. Before this, he had submitted to five attempts at surgical resection and radium treatment was instituted because of severe epistaxis. We have calculated that he was exposed to a mucosal dosage of at least 60,000 rads and believe that this induced the anaplastic carcinoma of the nasopharynx which killed him 40 years later. We believe that careful radiotherapy with a dose of 3000 rads in a three-week period is unlikely to produce any significant carcinogenic effect over the long term. We do not like to repeat radiotherapy, but in the presence of severe symptoms and massive, unresectable tumor, it is a lifesaving measure. Irradiation produces thrombosis and fibrosis with tumor regression and in our opinion, it is the treatment of choice for all but small tumors.

Although the endocrine status of these patients is indeterminate, our studies revealed no significant abnormalities. Our three female patients appeared normal in every way. Some authorities have recommended that these tumors be treated with hormones on the assumption that pituitary dysfunction is responsible for the growth of ectopic nasal erectile tissue[8,9]. Androgen therapy in two of our patients produced no detectable change, and we do not want to use estrogen in adolescent males because this may limit growth by inducing premature closure of the bony epiphysis.

The management recommended for these patients is summarized in Tables X and XI.

TABLE X

Recommended Management of Patients with Nasopharyngeal Angiofibroma

NASOPHARYNGEAL ANGIOFIBROMA

INVESTIGATIONS

History	X-ray - Skull +
	Coronal Tomograms
Clinical Examination	? Carotid Angiogram (s)
Nasopharynx	Laboratory - Blood
	Endocrine
Endocrine	Genetic

TABLE XI

Princess Margaret Hospital Treatment of Nasopharyngeal Angiofibroma

TREATMENT

Small Tumour Symptoms ± → Observation

Large Tumour Symptoms +++ → Radiation 3000 rads - 15 Rx - 3/52

↓

OBSERVATION AND PATIENCE

NO INTERFERENCE

Tumour Regression < Immediate / Delayed (up to 2 yrs.)

Residual Tumour (Asymptomatic) → No Rx

SUMMARY

Thirty-nine patients including three females with nasopharyngeal angiofibroma were seen at the Princess Margaret Hospital, Toronto, between 1946 and 1971. Thirty of 38 patients had bone destruction with extension into the air sinuses, orbit and cranium. It is important to treat the total tumor, and its many ramifications are best detected by coronal tomography. Radiotherapy should be sophisticated so as to treat the entire tumor volume while sparing normal structures. Three thousand rads in three weeks produces thrombosis, fibrosis and tumor regression, although up to two years may pass before it finally disappears. After irradiation, only six patients developed tumor recurrence; four of these required irradiation before the tumor finally disappeared.

ACKNOWLEDGEMENTS

These patients were investigated and treated by various members of the radiotherapy staff of the Princess Margaret Hospital and we are grateful to them for allowing us to describe their patients. Dr. J. W. Meakin advised on the endocrine assessment, Dr. T. C. Brown reviewed the microscopic slides and confirmed the diagnosis of angiofibroma. Dr. David Rideout produced the radiographs and developed the technique of coronal tomography as the optimum method for tumor assessment. Our thanks go to the Department of Medical Photography for preparation of figures and tables, and to Miss Pat Reeder for typing the manuscript.

REFERENCES

1 JEREB, Berta: Juvenile nasopharyngeal angiofibroma. *Acta Radiol [Ther] (Stockh)*, **9:** 302, 1970.

2 CONLEY, J., et al.: Nasopharyngeal angiofibroma in juvenile. *Surg Gynecol Obstet*, **126:** 825, 1968.

3 PIMPINELLA, R. J.: Nasopharyngeal angiofibroma in adolescent male. *J Pediatr*, **64:** 260, 1964.

4 APOSTOL, J. V. and FRAZELL, E. L.: Juvenile nasopharyngeal angiofibroma: Clinical Study. *Cancer*, **18:** 869, 1965.

5 THOMSEN, K. A.: Surgical treatment of juvenile nasopharyngeal angiofibroma. *Arch Otolaryngol*, **94:** 191, 1971.

6 FITZPATRICK, P. J.: Nasopharyngeal angiofibroma. *Clin Radiol*, **18:** 62, 1967.

7 FITZPATRICK, P. J.: The nasopharyngeal angiofibroma. *Can J Surg*, **13:** 228, 1970.

8 JOHNSEN, S., KLOSTER, J. H. and SCHIFF, M.: Action of hormones on juvenile nasophargyngeal angiofibroma: Case Report. *Acta Otolaryngol (Stockh)*, **61:** 153, 1966.

9 KARATAY, S. KATIRCIOGLU, S. and EROZDEN, O.: Significance of hormones in the pathogenesis of nasopharyngeal angiofibroma. *Acta Otolaryngol (Stockh)*, **56:** 1963.

RHABDOMYOSARCOMA IN CHILDHOOD

R. D. T. JENKIN, M.A., M.B., F.R.C.P.(C), F.F.R.*

Rhabdomyosarcoma is the commonest soft-tissue sarcoma of childhood (Table I). In a series of 101 consecutive children with soft-tissue sarcoma treated at the Princess Margaret Hospital during 1958-1970, 70 had rhabdomyosarcoma, and in a further 13 the diagnosis was unspecified sarcoma where the histological pattern was too poorly differentiated to permit further categorization. These 83 patients were all treated in the same fashion and will be analyzed together.

It is especially difficult to categorize a poorly differentiated sarcoma when the primary site of origin is paraspinal, related to the chest wall or is in the retroperitoneum (Table II). Differentiation from Ewing's sarcoma is especially difficult at these sites. In the paraspinal regions, neuroblastoma rarely causes difficulty in differential diagnosis because the abnormal pattern of excretion of catecholamine metabolites may readily be detected.

Table III shows the pattern of distribution by site of rhabdomyosarcoma in childhood. Tumors arising in the head and neck, and in the pelvis are the dominant groups in this series. Approximately 30% of our patients are alive with follow-up intervals ranging from 1-13 years.

TABLE I

Histological Distribution
101 Consecutive Children with Soft-Tissue Sarcoma

Soft Tissue Sarcoma Age < 16 yrs. PMH 1958 - 1970	
Rhabdomyosarcoma Inc. Malig. Mesenchymoma	70
Sarcoma Unspecified	13
Fibrosarcoma	10
Other Specific Sarcoma	8
	101

*The Princess Margaret Hospital, Toronto; and Assistant Professor of Radiology, University of Toronto.

TABLE II

Correlation of Histological Diagnosis and Anatomical Site of Primary Tumor

Rhabdomyosarcoma
Age < 16 yrs.
PMH 1958 - 1970

	Site	
	Chest Wall Spine Retroperitoneum	Other
Rhabdomyosarcoma Inc. Malig. Mesenchymoma	7	63
Sarcoma Unspecified	8	5

TABLE III

Distribution by Size of Rhabdomyosarcoma and Unclassified Soft-Tissue Sarcoma

Rhabdomyosarcoma
Age < 16 yrs.

Primary Site

	No. Patients	No. Alive
Head & Neck	31	10
Trunk	15	4
Pelvis & Genitalia	24	6
Limb	12	4
Bile Ducts	1	0
	83	24

The prospect for cure in rhabdomyosarcoma has improved in recent years as may be seen when we compare patients treated from 1958 to 1965, to those treated from 1966 to 1970 (Fig. 1). In the more recent group 50%, 13 of 26 patients, are alive at three years, compared to 21% for the earlier years. Whilst these are crude comparisons we could detect no obvious difference in the patients in the two groups. Both groups contained approximately 20% of patients with metastatic disease at diagnosis, the same proportions of patients in whom only a biopsy or partial excision of the tumor had been undertaken, and an equal number of patients with tumors at more favourable sites. Since patients are referred to the Princess Margaret Hospital for irradiation or chemotherapy, this is a select group which omits both ends of the spectrum. On the one hand it omits patients treated by a complete surgical procedure only, and on the other, it omits those with overwhelming disease, which prevented transfer to a specialist hospital.

When we compare, for these two time intervals, the survival curve and the curve demonstrating the proportion of patients free of metastatic or recurrent disease, we see that, for 1958-1965 (Fig. 2), recurrence took place usually in the first six months, and almost always within the first year after diagnosis. During 1966-1970, fewer patients had recurrences but the time of recurrence was very little changed (Fig. 3).

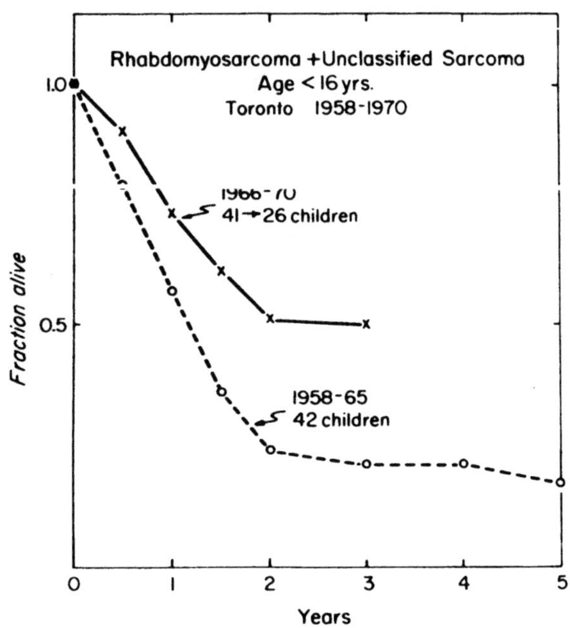

Fig. 1. Crude survival in children diagnosed during 1958-65, and during 1966-70.

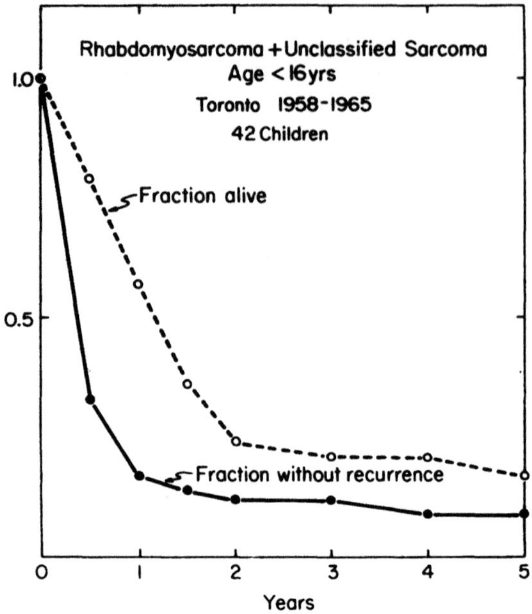

Fig. 2. A comparison of crude survival and recurrence-free survival – children treated during 1958-65.

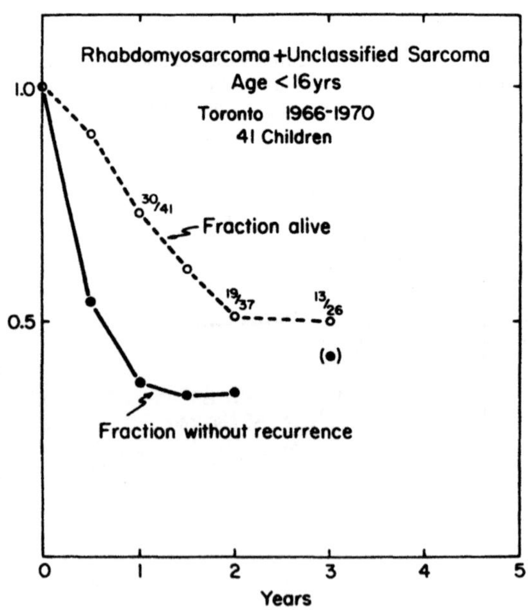

Fig. 3. A comparison of crude survival and recurrence-free survival – children treated during 1966-70.

TREATMENT VARIABLES

The manner in which these patients were treated changed during these years. All patients had undergone a surgical procedure, most often a simple biopsy, less often a partial removal and, occasionally, a complete excision, although in these latter cases we usually had grounds for believing that they had microscopic residual disease. Does the extent of the surgical procedure influence the cure rate? Table IV relates the extent of surgery to the number of patients alive and to the number dead, but separates those in whom the primary was controlled until death. It can be seen that control was more frequent if the tumor or part of the tumor had been removed. Thus, the primary remains controlled or was controlled until death in 14 of 24 patients subjected to a procedure in excess of biopsy, whereas control was achieved in only 15 of 40 patients who had only biopsy. The numbers available do not permit additional analysis by site, although, in general, it is the worst tumors in the least accessible sites which discourage the surgeon from doing any more than a biopsy. These results also make it quite clear that postoperative irradiation offers some chance for cure even when the surgical procedure is limited to biopsy.

The manner in which irradiation was given changed during the course of this study. In the early years, we employed modest-volume, modest-dose techniques and, in later years, generous-volume, high-dose techniques. When we compare tumor control with the relative volumes irradiated (Table V), we see that irradiation of a relatively small volume was associated with a small chance of controlling the tumor and *vice versa.*

Soft-tissue sarcomas are often much more extensive than palpation alone suggests. Therefore it is important to undertake a complete investigation of every patient to determine the anatomical extent of their disease and one should err on the side of treating too large a volume rather than too small, because if any part of a tumor is untreated local recurrence is assured.

The dose of irradiation used is illustrated for primary sites in the head, neck and limbs (Fig. 4). In 10 of 13 patients given high doses (below the line), the primary tumor was controlled either to the present or to the death of the patient, whereas primary control was achieved in only four of 13 patients at the lower doses represented above the line. The data for primary tumors of the orbit are shown separately (Fig. 5). In seven of 10 patients the higher doses represented beneath the line controlled the tumor. For tumors arising in the pelvis and trunk, lower doses of irradiation were used. Tumor control was obtained in five of 22 patients given these lower doses (Fig. 6 – above the line). Lower doses were used in these patients because of the large volume of tissue being irradiated and often because it was not anticipated that the treatment would have any but a palliative effect.

TABLE IV

Correlation of Extent of Operation and Control of Primary Site by Postoperative Irradiation

Rhabdomyosarcoma
Age <16 yrs.

Extent of Surgery	Alive	Dead	
	Primary Controlled	Primary Controlled	Primary Recurrent
B	6	9	25
P	3	0	6
MR	4	3	3
C	3	1	1
	26 - 120 mos.	3 - 56 mos.	

B - Biopsy
P - Partial excision
MR - Microscopic residual
C - Complete excision

TABLE V

Correlation of Relative Volume Irradiated with Control or Recurrence at Primary Site

Rhabdomyosarcoma
Age <16 yrs.

Primary Tumour Status	Relative Volume Irradiated		
	Large %	Medium %	Small %
Controlled (28 pts.)	64	29	7
Recurrent (33 pts.)	46	21	33

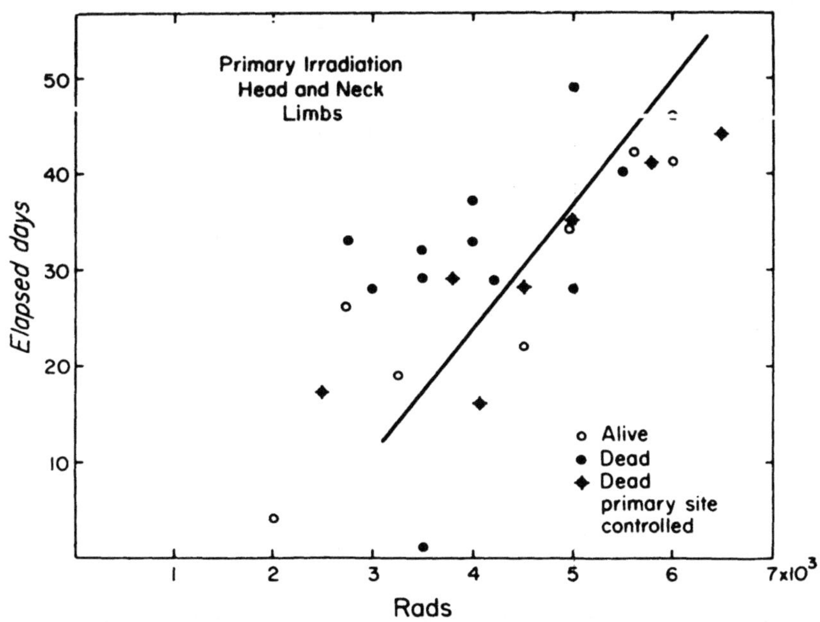

Fig. 4. Time/dose relationships for primary irradiation – head, neck and limb tumors.

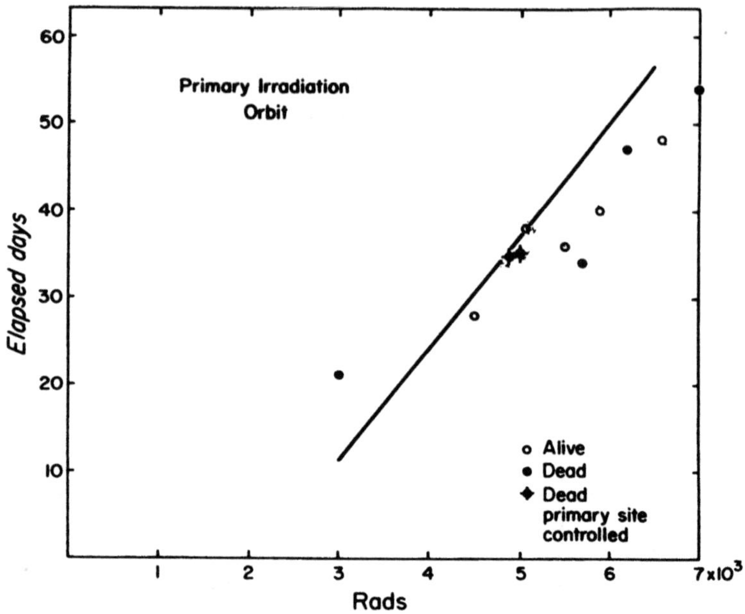

Fig. 5. Time/dose relationships for primary irradiation – orbital tumors.

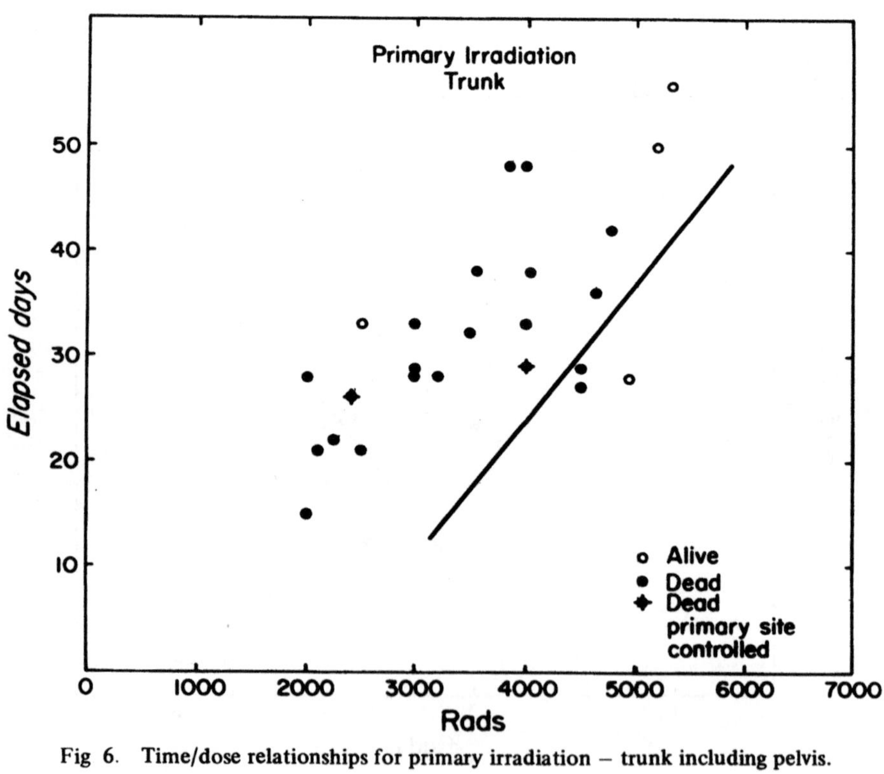

Fig 6. Time/dose relationships for primary irradiation – trunk including pelvis.

These dose-time data make it clear that, for a reasonable chance of permanent control in rhabdomyosarcoma, a high dose is necessary, certainly not less than 5000 rads in five weeks.

Appropriate surgery and irradiation without chemotherapy offers a fair chance of cure in rhabdomyosarcoma. In this series, of 24 surviving patients, 22 are trouble free and have a good chance for cure. Of these 24, only four received chemotherapy at any stage in their disease. Therefore, with regard to the final cure rate, these survival curves can be said to represent those obtainable with surgery and irradiation alone.

The manner in which irradiation is used for a solitary recurrence is also important. Of our 24 survivors, five were controlled after recurrence: one after recurrence at the primary site, two after the development of regional lymph nodes, one after development of a pulmonary metastasis, and one after development of a secondary lesion in a rib.

CHEMOTHERAPY

Over the years of this study, chemotherapy has become increasingly important. Actinomycin-D, vincristine and cyclophosphamide each have a good chance of inducing a remission in the metastatic phase of this disease. Until recently, we did not use chemotherapy electively, but reserved it for treatment of recurrence. Good palliation and useful prolongation of life was obtained with these agents. Thus, of 56 patients dying of metastatic rhabdomyosarcoma, 47 received chemotherapy and their survival ranged from one to 40 months from the time of their first recurrence, with an average survival of 10 months, and a median of nine months. In comparison, nine patients who received no chemotherapy survived one to five months, with an average of three months from the time of the first recurrence.

Whilst excellent remissions may be obtained with these agents used sequentially, late in the disease, cures are not obtained. However, evidence is building that the elective use of these agents in combination, particularly in the most favorable group of patients, where the surgical removal has been apparently complete and postoperative irradiation given, may appreciably increase the survival rate. Certainly this is true during the first two or three years following diagnosis and, for this reason, most of our patients now receive elective, maintained, combination chemotherapy with actinomycin-D, vincristine and cyclophosphamide. Whether we can justify the associated morbidity over the long term depends on whether the final cure rate is increased; this has not yet been determined.

SUMMARY

The maximum chance for cure in childhood rhabdomyosarcoma depends on adequate radical surgery or, for the majority where this is not possible, a lesser surgical procedure combined with irradiation to an adequate volume and to a dose of not less than 5000 rads in five weeks. Elective, maintained, combination chemotherapy improves the initial control rate and, hopefully, will produce higher final cure rates.

MALIGNANT LIVER TUMORS IN CHILDHOOD

SIGMUND H. EIN, M.D., F.R.C.S.(C) * and CLINTON A. STEPHENS, M.D., F.R.C.S.(C)**

Before 1960, few, if any, children with malignant liver tumors survived. However, reports of more aggressive investigation and treatment have recently appeared, and we are now beginning to achieve some encouraging results with these difficult and discouraging tumors of childhood.

The purpose of this paper is to review the records of 31 children with malignant tumors who received treatment at the Hospital for Sick Children, Toronto, between 1950 and 1971. This series does not include liver tumors discovered at post mortem examination.

CLINICAL MATERIAL

These 31 children with malignant tumors were evenly divided between both sexes. The youngest child with such a tumor was 10 weeks old. One quarter of all the malignant tumors were found in children less than one year of age and one-half of these were noted before five years of age.

The signs and symptoms were usually present for three months before discovery of the liver tumor; and every child with such a tumor presented with a hard upper abdominal mass. In one-half of the cases, this mass was the only sign or symptom of the disease. More than one-half the cases had upper abdominal pain. One-third of this group had added features, which seemed to accompany any malignancy in childhood – fever, malaise, anorexia, nausea, vomiting, weight loss, pallor and listlessness. Four children were jaundiced and two others had pre-existing cirrhosis, due to tyrosinemia and aminoaciduria.

In this group of children the results of hematological and biochemical tests were of no specific value. One-half of the children had hemoglobin concentration of less than 10 mg.%. The liver function tests in almost all cases (including the four jaundiced children) were within normal limits. A few had elevated alkaline phosphatase determinations. Platelet counts were obtained in almost every child with liver malignancy and only four were above 400,000. Alpha-1-fetal globulins measured in one child were positive.

*Staff Surgeon, Division of General Surgery, The Hospital for Sick Children, Toronto.

**Chief of General Surgery, The Hospital for Sick Children, Toronto.

Four of the 31 children presented with lung metastases which were seen on initial chest radiographs. One of these children also had metastases in each humerus. Another four had calcifications on plain abdominal films. The results of intravenous pyelography and gastrointestinal barium contrast studies were of some value in the investigation of malignant liver tumors in that they tended to rule out other intra-abdominal and retroperitoneal lesions. Three liver scans were obtained: one did not delineate a golf-ball sized lesion, although it was easily seen on arteriography. The latter study has been performed since 1967 in almost all children with liver cancer and it has proved the most rewarding of all investigations done to date. In all, seven arteriograms have been performed and, in two of the earlier studies, the incorrect diagnosis of neuroblastoma was made. However, in all subsequent cases, the diagnosis has been exact and correct.

PATHOLOGY, TREATMENT AND RESULTS

Of these 31 children, 28 had primary malignant liver tumors which fell into eight different pathological classifications (Table I). These diagnostic labels were assigned by a number of pathologists at the Hospital for Sick Children over a 10-year span and, in the near future, all this material will be reviewed by a single pathologist to determine if there is any correlation between the pathological type and the child's prognosis. Three children had secondary malignant tumors (two Wilms' and one malignant teratoma) – these are included because all presented as a primary liver malignancy.

TABLE I

Malignant Liver Tumors, 1950-1971

Primary		28
Carcinoma of liver		
Hepatoblastoma		
Hepatocholangioma		
Hepatoma		
Malignant cholangioma		
Malignant hepatoma		
Primary carcinoma of liver		
Primary liver cell carcinoma		
Secondary		3
Wilms'	2	
Teratoma	1	

The three common forms of treatment (surgery, radiotherapy, and chemotherapy) can be applied to these malignant liver tumors; however, as will be shown, only successful surgery is curative. On the 31 tumors operated on, 19 could only be biopsied. At operation each of these tumors was unresectable; in several cases, there were widespread metastases both in the liver and the abdomen. Of these biopsied patients, 75% received some form of postoperative therapy, which in all cases was palliative. Almost all received radiotherapy and one-half received some form of chemotherapy in addition. One patient received one month of intrahepatic arterial 5-FU which had no apparent effect. All five children who received no postoperative palliation, died within three months, most within the first week. Most of the 14 remaining children, who did receive some palliative treatment, lived several months before dying. Two of this group lived about one year after surgery.

The remaining 12 children who were operated on all had resections of a malignant liver tumor (Table II). Eight resections were for cure and no gross evidence of tumor was left behind. All but two of these children were under three and one-half years. The two children with large secondary Wilms' tumors were six and nine years old at the time of liver lobectomy. Seven of these eight patients who were operated on for cure are alive from one month up to 12 years after surgery. The only child who died in this group had five years of normal life before he developed lung metastases and symptoms. He died within two months in spite of chemotherapy. At post mortem, no tumor was found in his abdomen. Except for one of the two children with Wilms' tumor who had a secondary removed from his liver, none of these eight children had any other form of tumor therapy. Unfortunately the four children who had palliative resections all died in less than one year despite other therapy. Therefore, of these children with malignant liver disease, seven out of 31 have survived to date. Of those who have survived, all were under 11 years of age when the tumor was discovered.

TABLE II

Malignant Liver Tumors, 1950-1971
Resections

Curative		8
Survivors	7	
1 mo., 2,5,6,7,9,12 yr.		
Dead	1	
5 yr.		
Palliative		4
Survivors	0	
Dead	4	

DISCUSSION

All these children had hard upper abdominal masses when the tumor was discovered and all had signs and symptoms of their liver malignancy for three months which reflects the rapid growth of these malignant tumors. At least two-thirds of these children were in good general condition at the time of diagnosis[1].

The only laboratory test of any diagnostic value was the alpha-1-fetal globulins; this test, like VMA in determining neuroblastoma, is also valuable in following the course of malignant liver tumors. However, up to the present, this determination has been extremely difficult to obtain. We have not found any correlation between increased platelets and liver malignancy. In one child whose liver tumor was incompletely resected, the platelet count fell from 700,000 to less than 400,000!

We have been impressed with arteriography as a means of detecting and delineating these tumors; it is on this study that we now rely the most. Liver scans can miss small tumors.

The fact that only one-third of these lesions are resectable when discovered also strongly suggests their rapid growth. Although most of these tumors are more common in younger children, the overall resectability rate was only one-third. Other series[1] have reported a higher rate. Since we have observed, much to our dismay, recurrence in the form of lung metastases five years after a "curative" resection, we now consider that no patient is "cured" until he has lived tumor-free more than five years after resection. In our series, five of the seven survivors are in this happy category. It is also quite apparent that nothing short of a curative resection will cure the child with a liver malignancy and therefore the surgery must be aggressive. We have also encountered several children with large liver tumors, which were grossly malignant; however, after lobectomy and histological section, these were found to be benign hamartomas. In such cases resection is a wiser course than biopsy [2].

Our surgical approach to partial hepatectomy follows that laid down by many authors[3,4,5] – several intravenous "lines", hypothermia, abdomino-thoracic incision and so on. In one-half of our resections, the child's blood loss exceeded his blood volume. Intra-operative cardiac arrest occurred in four children; one of these died in the operating room. Such arrest seems to be more common in children than in adults, – an observation that has been made by others[3]. The children whose liver tumors were resected for cure had a fairly smooth postoperative course.

SUMMARY

Thirty-one children with malignant liver tumors have been treated at the Hospital for Sick Children, Toronto, between 1950 and 1971. One-quarter of these tumors were found in children less than one year of age, and one-half were found before five years. The signs and symptoms were usually present for three months and all patients had a hard upper abdominal mass. One-half of these children had abdominal pain. Arteriography was the best investigative tool. When resected for cure, the results were excellent. However, resectibility was feasible in only one-third of these children. Other forms of cancer therapy were of no value.

REFERENCES

1 LIN, T., CHEN, C. and LIU, W.: Primary carcinoma of the liver in infancy and childhood. *Surgery,* **60:** 1275, 1966.

2 CLATWORTHY, H. W., BOLES, E. T. and NEWTON, W. A.: Primary tumors of the liver in infants and children. *Arch Dis Child,* **35:** 22, 1960.

3 CLATWORTHY, H. W. and BOLES, E. T.: Right lobectomy of the liver in children. *Surgery,* **39:** May 1956.

4 PACK, G. T. and ISLAMI, A. H.: Operative treatment of hepatic tumors. *Ciba Clin Symp,* **16:** 38, 1964.

5 BRUNSCHWIG, A.. The surgery of hepatic neoplasms, with special reference to right and left hepatic lobectomies. *Cancer,* **6:** 725, 1953.

NEUROBLASTOMA

ODILE SCHWEISGUTH*

Of the malignant tumors in children, neuroblastoma is one in which no substantial therapeutic progress has been made in recent years. However, the unpredictability of its course and the possible contribution of immunological processes to its clinical course make it a fascinating disease.

The primary tumor develops at any site where embryonic sympathetic cells (neural crest cells) are located: two-thirds appear in the retroperitoneal area either from the adrenal medulla or the sympathetic ganglia, one-quarter in the posterior mediastinum and others in the cervical area, the pelvis, or the orbit. Very few are multiple: 1% of 400 children seen at Institut Gustave-Roussy. In some cases, the primary site is never found.

Neuroblastoma is the malignant tumor: ganglioneuroma is its mature, benign counterpart. The mixed tumor is the ganglioneuroblastoma. The tumor disseminates widely in many cases. Neuroblastoma is probably the most lymphophilic tumor in children. It spreads by the lymphatics to the retroperitoneal nodes, as may be shown by the intravenous pyelogram and can be confirmed by a lymphogram, then to the supraclavicular nodes. By the blood stream, the cells travel widely but grow mainly in the liver (chiefly in infants) and in the bone marrow, where extensive deposits are found only too frequently: on the contrary, pulmonary metastases are rare.

At the time of diagnosis, 60% of our patients have anemia and this is a bad prognostic sign[1]. This finding is not well correlated with bone involvement as determined by radiology, bone marrow smears and biopsy. While the anemia in most patients can be explained in terms of metastatic bone disease, in some no involvement of the bone can be demonstrated. The bone marrow of these patients shows prominent erythroblastosis (up to 70%) with macroblastosis and maturation arrest at the late stages. In a few cases studied with Fe^{59} and Cr^{51}, the results favored red-cell aplasia (in marked contrast to the rich cytology and histology of the bone marrow) associated with peripheral hemolysis. This phenomenon calls for further investigation.

Some neuroblastomas, mainly in infants, are detected because of a mass and the victim may have almost no symptoms.

The intravenous pyelogram is the best single investigation for retroperitoneal tumors: a neuroblastoma usually pushes the kidney and/or the ureter downwards or sideways. The calyces are not usually distorted. Displacement of the contralateral kidney is usually evidence of lymph-node extension.

*Service de Pediatrie, Institut Gustave-Roussy, Villejuif, France.

A chest film taken routinely during the investigation of common respiratory symptoms may lead to the discovery of an unsuspected posterior mediastinal tumor. Erosion of the ribs and calcification of the mass, which is present in about one-half of these children, makes the diagnosis of neurogenic tumor simpler. The physician must also look for enlargement of the intervertebral foramina and neurological deficit because of the occasional dumb-bell tumor with compression of the spinal cord[2].

Horner's syndrome may be associated either with apical thoracic tumors or with cervical tumors. In the latter, paralysis of the last cranial nerves may be present.

Pelvic tumors may often cause ureteric or rectal obstruction in small infants. The ureters can be severely compressed and produce ureterohydronephrosis. At rectal examination the tumor lies posterior and can be mistaken for a sacrococcygeal dysembryoma.

In all cases, the physician must seek evidence for extension of the disease and his studies will include a bone marrow "smear", radiographs of the skeleton and a search for invaded lymph nodes and subcutaneous metastases.

However, in two-thirds of all cases, neuroblastoma is discovered through symptoms produced by metastatic disease.

Bone metastases give rise to the most common picture, namely, exophthalmia with hematoma of the orbit, bone or articular pain, fever, anemia and loss of weight. The differential diagnosis includes rheumatic fever or, after the bone marrow examination, acute leukemia. An enlarged left supraclavicular node is sometimes the first sign. A complete investigation is then necessary to find the primary tumor.

Massive metastatic enlargement of the liver, Pepper's syndrome[3], is found only in infants younger than six months; in them, it is one of the most common causes of massive hepatomegaly.

Classically the primary tumor is found in the adrenal, but in three (10%) of our patients the primary was elsewhere: once in the neck, and twice in the mediastinum.

Sometimes subcutaneous metastases are found chiefly in babies. These may be numerous and often are associated with liver disease.

BIOCHEMISTRY

For 15 years it has been recognized that neuroblastoma cells can synthesize catecholamines[4]. Sometimes, the synthesis stops at the dopamine level and then homovanillic acid (HVA) is the main degradation product excreted in the urine. Usually noradrenaline is synthesized, but o-catecholmethyltransferase, present in the tumor cells, destroys this hypertensive substance. Methoxy-hydroxyphenyl-glycol (MHPG), which is produced in the tumor and released into the blood stream, is excreted in the urine as vanillyl mandelic acid (VMA)[5]. As a consequence, secreting neuroblastomas do not produce hypertension, as do pheochromocytomas, unless pressure on or obstruction of the renal vessels leads to hypertension by another mechanism.

In 90% of cases, an accurate diagnosis of neuroblastoma can be made, without histological proof, by an assay of urinary VMA and HVA. Quantitative evaluation requires two dimensional chromatography, but "spot-tests" have been described[6,7], which can be done at the bedside. These have to be controlled but, in tumors with a high rate of secretion, the spot test permits a quick diagnosis with a fairly good rate of confirmation. With these assays, surgical biopsy or exploratory laparotomy can be avoided, especially in patients with metastases, where these procedures are not indicated for therapeutic purposes. Often, biochemical investigation can be complemented by the cytological examination of aspirates from a metastatic lymph node and/or the bone marrow.

These biochemical assays are also useful during follow-up. After complete removal of the tumor, or successful chemotherapy or radiotherapy, urinary catecholamine levels are normal. Local relapse or distant metastases are usually signalled by an elevated excretion. However, in these instances, the type of excretion can differ from that observed previously: a non-excreting tumor can become highly secreting or *vice versa.*

Other substances such as cystathionine[8,9], homoserin[10], and N acetyl-tyramine[11], may also be found in excess in the urine.

SPECIAL SYNDROMES

Sympathetic tumors may be associated with certain apparently inappropriate clinical symptoms.

(a) *Chronic diarrhea* has been described in a number of children with neuroblastoma or ganglioneuroma since 1959[12,13]. The clinical picture mimics a celiac syndrome and the tumor will only be discovered after careful investigation: by radiological means in the thorax or the abdomen, and by searching for elevated excretion of catecholamines. Diarrhea stops as soon as the tumor is removed. To my knowledge, nothing is known concerning the substance secreted by the tumor and responsible for diarrhea.

(b) *Cushing's syndrome* has also been described in association with neuroblastoma[14,15,16]. Again the pathophysiology of this "paraneoplastic" disease is unknown. These two examples demonstrate how little we know of the biochemistry of neuroblastoma.

(c) *Opsomyoclonic Encephalopathy.* This syndrome, which has been delineated more recently, seems to be more common than previously thought. We have seen six examples of this among our 400 patients and more are being reported[17-23]. The neurological syndrome associated with neuroblastoma is called "acute cerebellar ataxia" or, better still, "opsomyoclonic encephalopathy", because it is not a cerebellar syndrome. In these cases, the evolution of the neurological symptoms and of the tumor can be completely independent: opsomyoclonies can appear long before the tumor can be diagnosed, at a time when there is no apparent cause for the child's complaint. Repeated radiological and biochemical investigations are necessary to detect the neuroblastoma, sometimes many months later. Resection of the tumor will not always alter the course of the neurological disease. Sometimes opsomyoclonies disappear and do not return with tumor recurrence or metastasis; sometimes the neuroblastoma is cured, but the encephalopathy continues for months or years and may seriously disturb the psychic development. Once again, we know nothing about the pathophysiology of this association which seems too frequent to occur only by chance.

TREATMENT

The results of treatment correlate strongly with the extent of disease at diagnosis[24,25].

Stages I and II

Localized disease is seen mainly in infants under one year of age, and in mediastinal tumors which are more frequently partially mature ganglioneuroblastomas than are tumors in the retroperitoneum.

Everybody agrees that primary treatment for such cases is surgery. Complete removal is often feasible: however, adhesions to the posterior wall or to the big vessels, or local nodal spread sometimes make complete resection difficult or dangerous and small "rests" of tumor may have to be left in place.

The value of adjuvant treatment is debatable. Cure may follow incomplete resection. A clinical trial would be needed to determine whether routine postoperative irradiation is of value. We believe radiotherapy to be unnecessary in small babies who have undergone a complete, or almost complete tumor excision. We advise irradiation after incomplete ablation and/or in the presence of lymph-node invasion, particularly in older children. In babies, the dose is kept low (2000-2500 rads), and in older children, in whom spontaneous regressions are less likely, we use up to 3500 rads. The same is true of systemic chemotherapy: we use it routinely for about six months, but we know that other groups don't. Comparison of results awaits a properly controlled study.

Stage III

In my opinion, Stage III is a local-regional stage very close to disseminated disease. Most of the time, if the tumor is very big and, especially, if large vessels are embedded in a mass of metastatic lymph nodes, surgical removal is usually impossible. Furthermore, even if the skill of the surgeon makes it feasible, distant lymph nodes, mainly supraclavicular, usually appear in the next few weeks, with or without metastatic bone disease.

Stage IV

No recent advance in therapy has improved the outlook in this generalized disease.

Surgery can sometimes get rid of the primary tumor but, in our experience, it doesn't change the child's prognosis. Metastases continue to flourish everywhere.

Radiotherapy has a very important palliative role: bone pain is relieved better by 650 to 850 rads twice in 48 hours than by any analgesic. Radiotherapy can relieve, for a while, intracranial hypertension or shrink symptomatic mediastinal disease. It cannot cure the disease because it is impossible to give tumoricidal doses everywhere.

Chemotherapy has not progressed very much. Cyclophosphamide and vincristine are still probably the most useful drugs[26-29]. Trials of daunomycin, methotrexate, bleomycin and procarbazine[30-33] have been disappointing in our own experience.

Incomplete remissions are often observed, and even a small number of complete clinical and biochemical remissions. They last usually a few weeks, at the best a few months and, on the whole, death occurs in six months to one year.

However, there are some exceptions to this rule.

Stage IV^S (Special)

It has been necessary to create a special Stage IV^S to include patients with metastases only in liver, bone-marrow and subcutaneous tissue. Roughly, this group corresponds to what is called Pepper's syndrome in small infants. Cure can be quite spontaneous, with no more treatment than good nursing[34]. In most of the cases a very "light" treatment is sufficient and here host reactions are the most important reasons for the cure. We avoid primary surgery in these cases, relying on the very VMA level in these infants for diagnosis.

We try to induce regression of the liver deposits with a small dose of radiation (1000 rads in 10 days). Then the child is watched, with the addition of alternating chemotherapy – vincristine and cyclophosphamide once a week, if appropriate, until the liver has regressed and the VMA is normal. Laparotomy is done at that time to remove the primary tumor and biopsy the liver. Both may show only sclerosis, without residual tumor cells. This change is almost constant in the liver, but foci of tumor cells frequently remain in the adrenal. Of 28 personal cases in this category who have been followed-up for at least 18 months, 16 are cured and 12 have died. Six died in the first days of hospitalization, literally overwhelmed by the growing tumor. Five died much later from bone metastases, which became apparent two to 15 months after diagnosis and were as incurable as the usual lesions in Stage IV. One (who had not been operated for the primary tumor) died from local abdominal recurrence discovered five years after the first treatment.

Other Unusual Types

Some children with radiologically demonstrable bone metastases have an unusual pattern of evolution. Seven of our cases seem to be cured after four to 10 years, but six of them were less than one year of age at the time of treatment.

One child is living 10 years after diagnosis: his tumor was unresectable and has been irradiated. A "second-look" laparotomy three years later showed persistent tumor in the lymph nodes of the mesentery and around the appendix. Since that time, his VMA and HVA have been permanently elevated, despite all attempts at chemotherapy. However, the patient is well, without any clinical sign of disease.

Six children died finally of disseminated disease but after abnormally long delays[35] up to 10 years; one baby had spontaneous remission of extensive bone metastases for three years.

"Spontaneous" cures have often been attributed to maturation of the neuroblastoma to ganglioneuroma[36]. This can occur, but it is rare and difficult to demonstrate. It seems that the neuroblastoma cells are destroyed, at least in most children with liver metastases, because we have never found a single ganglion cell in biopsies made after regression of the tumor.

CONCLUSION

There are "good" neuroblastomas: localized or Stage IV^S (special) disease. For them, treatment must be light, surgical if possible and careful; the danger here is overtreatment of patients who are almost able to cure themselves. These patients are almost all less than one year of age.

There are "bad" neuroblastomas, Stages III and IV, for whom effective treatment is still to be found. Nevertheless, once in a while, one patient is unexpectedly cured, and we don't know why.

What are our hopes for the future? I don't expect much improvement in present methods and drugs. But we, as clinicians, should turn the research workers in a different direction: immunological processes, in the broadest sense of the term, will have to be thoroughly studied[37,38], with the hope, one day, of finding a clinical application. Nerve growth factor, if better purified, or an antiserum to this factor, is another possible approach[39], or the search for other antagonists of embryonic sympathetic cell growth[40].

REFERENCES

1 VIEU, F.: Contribution a l'étude de l'anemie du neuroblastome de l'enfant. Thése Universite; Paris Sud, 1971.

2 LEPINTRE, J., SCHWEISGUTH, O., LABRUNE, M. and LEMERLE, J.: Les neuroblastomes en sablier. Etude de 22 cas. *Arch Fr Pediatr,* **26:** 829, 1969.

3 PEPPER, W.: A study of congenital sarcoma of the liver and suprarenal. *Am J Med Sci,* **121:** 287, 1901.

4 BOHUON, C., ed: Neuroblastomas – Biochemical Studies. *In:* Recent Results in Cancer Research, Vol. 2, New York, Springer-Verlag, 1966.

5 LABROSSE, E. H.: Catechol-0-methyltransferase activity in neuroblastoma tumour. *Nature,* **196:** 1222, 1962.

6 EVANS, A. E., BLORE, J., HADLEY R. and TANINDI, S.: The Las Brosse spot test: A practical aid in the diagnosis and management of children with neuroblastoma. *Pediatrics,* **47:** 913, 1971.

7 GITLOW, S. E., BERTANI, L. M., RAUSEN, A., GRIBETZ, D. and DZIEDZIC, S. W.: Diagnosis of neuroblastoma by qualitative and quantitative determination of catecholamine metabolites in urine. *Cancer,* **25:** 1377, 1970.

8 GEISER, C. F. and EFRON, M. L.: Cystathioninuria in patients with neuroblastoma or ganglioneuroblastoma. Its correlation to vanilmandelic acid excretion and its value in diagnosis and therapy. *Cancer,* **22:** 856, 1968.

9 STUDNITZ, W. von: Cystathioninuria in children with neuroblastoma with and without metastasis. *Acta Paediatr Scand,* **59:** 80, 1970.

10 STUDNITZ, W. von: Homoserine in urine in patients with neuroblastoma. *Scand J Clin Lab Invest,* **17:** 558, 1965.

11 STUDNITZ, W. von and HANSON, A.: Demonstration of urinary N-acetyltyramine in patients with neuroblastoma. *Clin Chim Acta,* **16:** 180, 1967.

12 GREEN, M., COOKE, R. E. and LATTANZI, W.: Occurrence of chronic diarrhea in three patients with ganglioneuromas. *Pediatrics,* **23:** 951, 1959.

13 STICKLER, G. B., HALLENBECK, G. A., FLOCK, E. V. and ROSEVEAR, J. W.: Ganglioneuroblastoma and diarrhea. *Am J Dis Child,* **104:** 598, 1962.

14 KENNY, F. M., STAVRIDES, A., VOORHESS, M. L. and KLEIN, R.: Cushing's syndrome associated with an adrenal neuroblastoma. A case in an infant with clinical, pathological, and adrenal cortical and medullary hormone excretion studies. *Am J Dis Child,* **113:** 611, 1967.

15 KOGUT, M. D. and DONNELL, G. N.. Cushing's syndrome in association with renal ganglioneuroblastoma. *Pediatrics,* **28:** 566, 1961.

16 NORMANN, T., HAUNEN, J. and MJOLNEROD, O.: Cushing's syndrome in an infant associated with neuroblastoma in two ectopic adrenal glands. *J Pediatr Surg,* **6:** 197, 1971.

17 FOURNIER, A., PAULI, A.. DUCOULOMBIER, H.. COUSIN, J. and CARTON, M. B.: Syndrome oculo-cerebello-myoclonique et sympathoblastome. (A propos d'une observation). *Arch Fr Pediatr,* **27:** 766, 1970.

18 KOROBKIN, M., CLARK, R. E. and PALUBINSKAS, A. J.: Occult neuroblastoma and acute cerebellar ataxia in childhood. *Radiology,* **102:** 151, 1972.

19 LARBRE, F., BETHENOD, M., GUIBAUD, P., MAMELLE, J. C. and GENOUD, J.: Syndrome oculo-cerebello-myoclonique et neuroblastome. A propos de deux observations. *Arch Fr Pediatr,* **29:** 421, 1972.

20 LEMERLE, J., LEMERLE, M., AICARDI, J., MESSICA, C. and SCHWEISGUTH, O.: Trois cas d'association à un neuroblastome d'un syndrome oculo-cerebello-myoclonique. *Arch Fr Pediatr,* **26:** 547, 1969.

21 LEONIDAS, J. C., BRILL, C. B. and ARON, A.M.: Neuroblastoma presenting with myoclonic encephalopathy. *Radiology,* **102:** 87, 1972.

22 MARTIN, E. S., GRIFFITH, J. F. and DURHAM, N. C.: Myoclonic encephalopathy and neuroblastoma. *Am J Dis Child,* **122:** 257, 1971.

23 MOE, P. G. and NELLHAUS, G.: Infantile polymyoclonia-opsoclonuc syndrome and neural crest tumors. *Neurology (Minneap),* **20:** 756, 1970.

24 EVANS, A. E., D'ANGIO, G. J. and RANDOLPH, J.: A proposed staging for children with neuroblastoma. *Cancer,* **27:** 374, 1971.

25 KOOP, C. E. and JOHNSON, D. G.: Neuroblastoma: An assessment of therapy in reference to staging. *J Pediatr Surg,* **6:** 595, 1971.

26 EVANS, A. E., HEYN, R. M.. NEWTON, W. A. and LEIKIN, S. L.: Vincristine sulfate and cyclophosphamide. *JAMA,* **207:** 1325, 1969.

27 PINKEL, D., PRATT, C., HOLTON, C., JAMES, D., WRENN, E. and HUSTU, O.: Survival of children with neuroblastoma treated with combination therapy. *J Pediatr,* **73:** 928, 1968.

28 SAWITSKY, A., et al.: Vincristine and cyclophosphamide therapy on generalized neuroblastoma: A collaborative study. *Am J Dis Child,* **119:** 308, 1970.

29 WINDMILLER, J., BERRY, D. H. HADDY, T. B., VIETTI, T. J. and SUTOW, W. W.: Vincristine sulfate in the treatment of neuroblastoma in children. *Am J Dis Child,* **111:** 75, 1966.

30 FERNBACH, D. J., HADDY, T. B. HOLCOMB, T. M., STUCKEY, W. J., SULLIVAN, M. P. and WATKINS, W. L.: L-Sarcolysin (NSC-8806) therapy for children with metastatic neuroblastoma. *Cancer Chemother Rep,* **52:** 293, 1968.

31 FERNBACH, D. J., HADDY, T. B., HOLCOMB, T. M., LUSHER, J., SUTOW, W. W. and VIETTI, T. J.: Uracil mustard (NSC-34462) therapy for children with metastatic neuroblastoma. *Cancer Chemother Rep,* **52:** 287, 1968.

32 SAMUELS, L. D., NEWTON, W. A. and HEYN, R.: Daunorubicin therapy in advanced neuroblastoma. *Cancer,* **27:** 831, 1971.

33 SUTOW, W. W., FERNBACH, D. J., THURMAN, W. G., HOLTON, C. P. and WATKINS, W. L.: Daunomycin in the treatment of metastatic neuroblastoma. *Cancer Chemother Rep,* **54:** 283, 1970.

34 BODIAN, M.: Neuroblastoma. *Pediatr Clin North Am,* **6:** 449, 1959.

35 VOGEL, J. M., CODDON, D. R., SIMON, N. and GITLOW, S. E.: Osseous metastases in neuroblastoma. A 17-year survival. *Cancer,* **26:** 1354, 1970.

36 GOLDMAN, R. L., WINTERLING, A. N. and WINTERLING, C. C.: Maturation of tumours of the sympathetic nervous system. Report of long term survival in two patients, one with disseminated osseous metastases, and review of cases from the literature. *Cancer,* **18:** 1510, 1965.

37 BILL, A. H. and MORGAN, A.: Evidence for immune reactions to neuroblastoma and future possibilities for investigation. *J Pediatr Surg,* **5:** 111, 1970.

38 HELLSTROM, I. E., HELLSTROM, K. E., PIERCE, G. E. and BILL, A. H.: Demonstration of cell-bound and humoral immunity against neuroblastoma cells. *Proc Natl Acad Sci USA,* **60:** 1231, 1968.

39 KUMAR, S., STEWARD, J. K., WAGHE, M., PEARSON, D.. EDWARDS, D. C., FENTON, E. L. and GRIFFITH, A. H.: The administration of the nerve growth factor to children with widespread neuroblastoma. *J Pediatr Surg,* **5:** 18, 1970.

40 ANGELETTI, P. U. and LEVI-MONTALCINI, R.: Cytolytic effect of 6-hydroxy-dopamine on neuroblastoma cells. *Cancer Res,* **30:** 2863, 1970.

IMMUNOLOGICAL ASPECTS OF NEUROBLASTOMA

PETER B. DENT, M.D. *

Neuroblastoma has attracted the interest of oncologists and immunologists because it has a number of biological properties, which may provide some insight into the neoplastic process and the host's antitumor defense mechanisms. These features which have recently been reviewed[1], include an unusually high incidence of spontaneous regression. On the basis of autopsy studies of adrenal glands taken from infants dying from other causes, it has been calculated that the incidence of neuroblastoma *in situ* exceeds that of clinically diagnosed neuroblastoma by almost 100 fold. It has been postulated that some host control mechanism is responsible for this phenomenon. It is not yet clear whether this disparity is due to some sort of differentiative influence through which neuroblastomas can differentiate into benign ganglioneuromas; however, it has been recognized for several years that human neuroblastoma can display evidence of maturation when cultivated *in vitro*[2]. Recently, Schubert *et al.*[3] have shown that suitable modifications of culture conditions can reversibly alter the transplantable murine neuroblastoma from a typical neuroblast to a cell with neurite outgrowth resembling a more mature nerve cell. Whether there is an accompanying change in the malignant behavior of such cells is not known. Further studies in this system are urgently needed to determine whether induction of differentiation in a neoplastic cell might control the malignant process.

That immunological factors may be involved in control of human neuroblastoma has only recently been appreciated. Evidence suggesting that this is so has come from the observations that lymphocyte infiltration is more common in tumors which carry a more favorable prognosis[4] and that patients with a high peripheral lymphocyte count seem to do better than patients with a low lymphocyte count[5]. With neuroblastoma as with other solid tumors, patients who develop delayed hypersensitivity reactions in response to topical sensitization with dinitrochlorobenzene have a more favorable prognosis[6]. The studies of Hellstrom and others, which will be discussed in detail below, give more direct evidence that specific antitumor immunity plays a role in neuroblastoma.

*Department of Pediatrics, McMaster University, Hamilton, Ontario.

TUMOR ANTIGENS AND ANTITUMOR IMMUNITY

The concept of antitumor immunity is predicated on the existence of tumor-specific antigens[7]. Essentially, these are antigens, which are present on tumor cells but are not detected on the normal tissues from which the tumors arise. Animal studies indicate that, in general, there are two types of tumor antigens – those associated with virus-induced tumors which, for any given virus, are identical in any species or tissue type, and those associated with chemical carcinogens, which are usually individually distinct, i.e., the same carcinogen given in two sites to the same animal can give rise to two tumors with different tumor-specific antigens. While tumor antigens may be found in the nucleus or cytoplasm of the cell, or may be associated with a specific product of the cell, the most important tumor antigens are found on the cell surface. These, the tumor-specific transplantation antigens, behave in the same way as histocompatibility antigens, in that they induce the rejection response by which the host suppresses the neoplastic process.

The antitumor immune response is of two main types – that which involves sensitized or "killer" lymphocytes, and that which involves serum antibody. The latter may defend the host against malignant cells by promoting phagocytosis of the tumor cells, or it may lyse the tumor cell by activating the complement system. Recent studies indicate that, in certain situations, patients with cancer have a serum factor, which blocks the killing effect of sensitized lymphocytes against tumor cells *in vitro*[8]. Sjogren and his colleagues have suggested that this factor may be an antibody that does not fix complement, or a complex of antibody with tumor antigen[9]. The clinical significance of this factor will be discussed later in connection with the data on tumor immunity in neuroblastoma.

Antitumor immunity has been measured by a wide variety of immunological techniques[7,10] which makes difficult the interpretation and collation of these data. However, this discussion will present only the techniques that have been used in studies on patients with neuroblastoma.

ANTITUMOR IMMUNITY IN HUMAN NEUROBLASTOMA

The pioneering work in this malignancy was done by the Hellstrom team, who demonstrated cell-mediated immunity and serum-blocking factors, using a technique in which cultured human neuroblastoma cells were the target antigen. Excised tumors are dissociated and placed into dishes to which lymphocytes from various donors are added. The tumor cells normally form colonies which can be counted after three to five days growth. Addition of immune lymphocytes reduces the number of these colonies presumably due to lymphocyte-mediated destruction of the tumor cells. As controls, normal skin fibroblasts derived from the same patient are used as target cells. To test for blocking factors, the cultured target cells are pretreated with test serum before addition of killer lymphocytes. When blocking factors are present, colony reduction decreases. In a few cases, cytotoxic antibodies were demonstrated by adding test plasma containing active complement to cultured tumor cells. The observations of the Hellstroms[11,12] can be summarized as follows:

Six out of six patients had cytotoxic lymphocytes when tested on their own cultured tumors;

Fourteen out of 16 patients had cytotoxic lymphocytes against allogeneic tumors. The intensity of the reaction appeared to be similar in both autochthonous and allogeneic combinations;

Cytotoxic lymphocytes were present in patients who were symptom free and those who had progressive disease;

Twelve of 16 mothers had cytotoxic lymphocytes when tested against neuroblastoma cells from their own children or other children. A large number of healthy siblings and parents also reacted positively;

The following specificity controls were always negative:

(a) patients' lymphocytes against skin fibroblasts or other tumor cells
(b) lymphocytes from normal donors against neuroblastoma cells
(c) lymphocytes from patients with other tumors against neuroblastoma cells

(occasionally a weak response was seen in the last instance.)

Six out of six patients with progressively growing neuroblastomas had serum-blocking factors while none of four "apparently cured" patients had such factors;

Three of six patients and four of four mothers had cytotoxic antibodies in their plasma.

Using a slightly different technique which still depends on the *in vitro* destruction of target neuroblastoma cells by killer lymphocytes, Jagarlamoody *et al.*[13] demonstrated cytotoxic lymphocytes in two patients with Heuioblastoma and blocking factois in one of them.

Finally, Kumar *et al.*[14] did lymphocyte cytotoxicity assays in eight patients with neuroblastoma using cell cultures derived from 11 neuroblastomas. They found a significant reduction in individual cell numbers in all patients with neuroblastoma. The difference between the killing activity of the patients' lymphocytes and normal control lymphocytes was not great; however, it was statistically significant. These workers found that the killing effect was specific in that it was always less on normal cells or unrelated tumor cells than on the neuroblastoma cells. Thus, while these data confirm the presence of both specific lymphocyte cytotoxicity and blocking antibody in patients with neuroblastoma, the presence and intensity of these responses have not been correlated with clinical parameters to determine whether they have any prognostic significance.

These observations appear to indicate the existence of a tumor-specific antigen in human neuroblastoma, and suggest that the antigen is common to all neuroblastomas and, therefore, resembles the virus-induced tumors of experimental animals. In this connection, a virus-like agent has been recovered from the transplantable murine neuroblastoma, which can induce *de novo* neuroblastomas in secondary hosts[15]. A transmissible agent in human neuroblastoma is suggested by the finding that mothers of patients with this tumor and other family members have demonstrable cellular and humoral immunity to the neuroblastoma antigen.

We still cannot be certain that there is a common neuroblastoma antigen because careful antigenic analyses have not yet been performed. Using the fluorescent antibody assay in patients with melanoma, Lewis *et al.*[16] have shown that there is a common cytoplasmic antigen but also that there is an individually specific cell-surface antigen. This point has some practical significance because, if each tumor has its own antigenic specificity, then all immunologic tests would have to be performed on the patient's own tumor thereby precluding large-scale diagnostic and prognostic tests. Fortunately, the current evidence from three separate studies of neuroblastoma patients points toward a common antigen in this neoplasm.

The presence of cytotoxic lymphocytes in all patients, regardless of their clinical status, is somewhat disturbing because it undermines the importance of this immune mechanism in the control of the tumor. However, it must be pointed out that no real quantitative studies of this response are available. Recently, O'Toole *et al.*[17] have shown that, by varying the lymphocyte-target cell ratio, they achieved some degree of quantitation, i.e., lower lymphocyte-to-target-cell ratios reflect more intense cell-mediated immunity. This correlation has not been examined in neuroblastoma patients.

The finding of blocking factors in the serum of patients with progressive tumors would explain the above paradox if such blocking factors were active *in vivo.* They are present *in vivo* in other systems as they have been eluted from actively growing tumors[18]. If the clinical correlations, which have been described by the Hellstroms, are confirmed, the assay of serum-blocking activity may become a useful way to monitor the progress of this disease.

Recent studies in other human tumor systems indicate that tumor-free patients have a serum factor, which "cancels" the blocking activity present in the serum of patients with progressively growing tumors[19]. However, we have no evidence of such a factor in tumor-free patients who have been successfully treated for neuroblastoma.

We appear to have at hand a possible means of obtaining more precise information on the delicate balance between tumor growth and host control mechanisms. Unfortunately, current assay methods are difficult to perform routinely. They require growing tumor cells usually in early passage. No results with established lines have been reported although such lines do exist[20].

Established lines have been used successfully in other tumor systems[17]. The killing reactions are difficult to quantitate and the problems of nonspecific killing and the use of inappropriate controls have thwarted many investigators who have pursued similar studies.

SUMMARY

It is now well recognized that some host mechanism may play a role in controlling the development and dissemination of neuroblastoma. The recent definition of tumor-specific antigens in human neoplasms and the discovery that tumor-bearing host responds immunologically to these antigens have stimulated a search for this response in patients with neuroblastoma. Preliminary results indicate that these patients have both cytotoxic lymphocytes and antibodies as well as a serum factor which inhibits lymphocyte cytotoxicity *in vitro*. There is also a suggestion that the blocking factor, which has also been termed "enhancing antibody", may be associated with a poor prognosis.

Before assays of anti-tumor immunity can be used more widely, we need more information on the tumor specific antigens of neuroblastoma; on the type and intensity of the response to these antigens, and on the clinical correlates of the immune response. Nevertheless, it appears at this time that quantitative, *in vitro* measurements of cell-mediated and humoral anti-tumor immunity may serve not only as indices of the completeness of surgical excision and of subsequent tumor recurrence, but as a guide for chemotherapy and immunotherapy.

REFERENCES

1 HELLSTROM, K. E. and HELLSTROM, I.: Immunity to neuroblastomas and melanomas. *Annu Rev Med*, **23:** 19, 1972.

2 MURRAY, M. R. and STOUT, A. P.: Distinctive characteristics of the sympathicoblastoma cultivated *in vitro*. A method for prompt diagnosis. *Am J Pathol*, **23:** 429, 1947.

3 SCHUBERT, D., HUMPHREYS, S., deVITRY, F. and JACOB, F.: Induced differentiation of neuroblastoma. *Dev Biol*, **25:** 514, 1971.

4 MARTIN, R. F. and BECKWITH, J. B.: Lymphoid infiltrates in neuroblastomas, their occurrence and prognostic significance. *J Pediatr Surg*, **3:** 161, 1968.

5 BILL, A. H. and MORGAN, A.: Evidence for immune reactions to neuroblastoma and future possibilities for investigation. *J Pediatr Surg*, **5:** 111, 1970.

6 HELSON, L., RAMOS, C. OETTGEN, H. and MURPHY, M.: DNCB reactivity in children with neuroblastoma. *Proc Am Assoc Cancer Res*, **12:** 86, 1971.

7 SMITH, R. T.: Tumor specific immune mechanisms. *New Engl J Med*, **278:** 1207, 1268, 1326, 1968.

8 HELLSTROM, K. E. and HELLSTROM, I.. Immunological enhancement as studied by cell culture techniques. *Annu Rev Microbiol*, **24:** 373, 1970.

9 SJOGREN, H. O., HELLSTROM, I., BANSAL, S. C. and HELLSTROM, K. E.: Suggestive evidence that the "blocking antibodies" of tumor-bearing individuals may be antigen-antibody complexes. *Proc Natl Acad Sci*, **68:** 1372, 1971.

10 COHEN, A. M. BURDICK, J. F. and KETCHAM, A. S.: Tumor specific cellular immunity. *J Surg Res*, **11:** 421, 1971.

11 HELLSTROM, I., HELLSTROM, K. E. BILL, A. H. PIERCE, G. E. and YANG, J. P. S.: Studies on cellular immunity to human neuroblastoma cells. *Int J Cancer,* **6:** 172, 1970.

12 HELLSTROM, I., HELLSTROM, K. E., PIERCE, G. E. and BILL, A. H.: Demonstration of cell-bound and humoral immunity against neuroblastoma cells. *Proc Natl Acad Sci,* **60:** 1231, 1968.

13 JAGARLAMOODY, S. M., AUST, J. C., TEW, R. H. and McKHANN, C. F.: *In vitro* detection of cytotoxic cellular immunity against tumor-specific antigens by a radioisotopic technique. *Proc Natl Acad Sci,* **68:** 1346, 1971.

14 KUMAR, S., TAYLOR, G., STEWARD, J. K., WAGHE, M. A. and PEARSON, D.: Cellular immunity in Wilms' tumor and neuroblastoma. *Int J Cancer,* **10:** 36, 1972.

15 PRASAD, K. N., ZAMBERNARD, J., LASHER, R. and VANWOERT, M. H.: Transmission of mouse neuroblastoma by a cell-free extract. *Nature,* **228:** 997, 1970.

16 LEWIS, M. G., IKONOPISOV, R. L., NAIRN, R. C., PHILLIPS, T. M., FAIRLEY, G. H., BODENHAM, D. C. and ALEXANDER, P.: Tumor-specific antibodies in human malignant melanoma and their relationship to the extent of disease. *Br Med J,* **3:** 547, 1969.

17 O'TOOLE, C. PERLMANN, P., ONSGAARD, B., MOBERGER, G. and EDSMYR, F.: Cellular immunity to human urinary bladder carcinoma. 1. Correlation to clinical stage and radiotherapy. *Int J Cancer,* **10:** 77, 1972.

18 SJOGREN, H. O., HELLSTROM, I., BANSAL, S. C., WARNER, G. A. and HELLSTROM, K. E.: Elution of "blocking factors" from human tumors, capable of abrogating tumor cell destruction by specifically immune lymphocytes. *Int J Cancer,* **9:** 274, 1972.

19 HELLSTROM, I., HELLSTROM, K. E., SJOGREN, H. O. and WARNER, G. A.: Serum factors in tumor-free patients cancelling the blocking of cell-mediated tumor immunity. *Int J Cancer,* **8:** 185, 1972.

20 TUMILOWICZ, J. J., NICHOLS, W. W., CHOLON, J. J. and GREENE, A. E.: Definition of a continuous human cell line derived from neuroblastoma. *Cancer Res,* **30:** 2110, 1970.

OPERATIVE TREATMENT OF NEUROBLASTOMA AND RHABDOMYOSARCOMA

C. EVERETT KOOP, M.D., Sc.D.*

NEUROBLASTOMA

Several widely-held concepts concerning the management of neuroblastoma have been changed radically, or at least slightly altered, since Evans, D'Angio and Randolph[1] proposed the staging scheme in 1971. The staging system we use at the Children's Hospital, Philadelphia, is outlined later in this paper.

Until then we accepted as truth that: the prognosis in neuroblastoma was better in children under one year of age as compared with older children; the site of origin of a given tumor had a definite relationship to survival; and the histological gradation of the tumor (from the highly malignant to the almost benign) was generally, but not always specifically, correlated with survival.

Although I had few supporters, I always believed that radiation therapy *per se* had little effect on the survival of patients with neuroblastoma, and in the management of my patients[2-5] I relied on aggressive, extirpative surgery rather than adjunctive therapy. I believed that the patient's own immune response or some other unknown mechanism caused residual tumor either to disappear or to mature, and I persisted in extirpative surgery only because no other reported methods of therapy produced better survival.

The role of operative treatment can be reviewed by referring to resectable, non-resectable, and metastatic disease, although so many variables operate in this disease that a protocol is difficult to establish.

We have managed 164 neuroblastomas, 150 of them with follow-up ranging from two to more than 20 years. The first 134 of these neuroblastomas form the basis of this discourse.

Resectable Tumors

There is no doubt that resectable tumors should be completely excised, although we have never advocated *en bloc* dissection of contiguous viscera. I believe that if the objective is to cleanly resect the tumor, operative removal should be the sole therapy, particularly in the child under one year of age. In our clinic at the Children's Hospital, these patients are never given radiation therapy, although we are now co-operating in a national study of postoperative chemotherapy.

---

*Surgeon-in-Chief, Children's Hospital of Philadelphia; and Professor of Pediatric Surgery, University of Pennsylvania.

Non-Resectable Tumors

If a tumor is deemed non-resectable by all clinical assessment available before operation, our plan of attack depends upon the presence or absence of bone metastases. It is most unusual to salvage a patient with neuroblastoma if he has demonstrable bone metastases (only one in our series). Therefore, if the tumor seems to be non-resectable and the child has evident bone metastases, we treat him by concomitant radiation (about 1200 r) and chemotherapy. The diagnosis can usually be made on the basis of radiographs, and by biochemical and histologic procedures, namely, by assessment of urinary catecholamines and by examination of the bone marrow. Then, six to eight weeks after radiation therapy, we explore the child and resect his primary tumor as completely as possible. In most cases, radiation therapy has been administered to metastatic lesions in the interim.

If tumor resectability can be assessed only after opening the chest or abdomen, in particularly hazardous situations such as an extremely vascular tumor or one which has wrapped about major vessels, we might "back out" after doing the biopsy and proceed with the therapy outlined above when we had a working preoperative diagnosis of non-resectability. On the other hand, if it were deemed safe, we would probably resect as much of the tumor as possible, usually after ligating as much of its arterial blood supply as we could. Neuroblastomas usually have a pseudocapsule and, in the abdomen, are often gelatinous under a rim of relatively firm tumor. When we find such a lesion, we spoon out the relatively liquid tumor (or suck it out), excise as much of the solid tumor as possible and then control the bleeding by mattress sutures. Although bleeding is frequently brisk, we have not yet seen a patient's life threatened by hemorrhage. Obviously, this sort of extirpation must be undertaken gingerly, and the surgeon should not make long sweeping incisions into vascular tumors until he has assessed the degree of vascularity.

Management of Non-Bony Metastases

Except for palpable lymph nodes in certain areas and malignant cells in the bone marrow, most non-bony metastases are not recognized until operation. In general, the presence of such metastatic spread does not affect the approach to the primary tumor, outlined above. The accessible, easily resectable metastatic spread in lymph nodes is extirpated. Because the behavior of these tumors depends upon so many factors other than the mode of surgical attack, we do not resect liver lobes or even bowel to remove metastatic nodes from the supporting mesentery.

Does Removal of the Primary Affect Metastases?

Although this question has not received a satisfactory answer, we believe that the primary lesion should be resected even though there are bony metastases and even if we have no assurance that such resection will affect these metastases. Our concept of partial resection (when total extirpation is impossible) derives from our early experience which seemed to show that patients so treated had a better survival rate than those who had only biopsies. This impression still remains, but we now have an additional reason for partial resection: the fewer the tumor cells left in the patient, the better chance he has for a favorable response to his own immune response and/or to chemotherapy.

The staging scheme mentioned above is shown in Table I.

TABLE I

Stage I:	Tumors confined to the organ or structure of origin.
Stage II:	Tumors extending in continuity beyond the organ or structure of origin but not crossing the midline. Regional lymph nodes on the homolateral side may be involved. (For tumors arising in the midline structures such as the organs of Zuckerkandl, penetration beyond the capsule and involvement of lymph nodes on the same side should be considered Stage II. Bilateral extension of any sort should be considered Stage III.)
Stage III:	Tumors extending in continuity beyond the midline. Regional lymph nodes may be involved bilaterally.
Stage IV:	Remote disease involving skeleton, organs, soft tissues, distant lymph-node groups, etc.
Stage IV^S:	Patients who would otherwise be Stage I or Stage II but who have remote disease confined to one or more of the following sites: liver, skin, or bone marrow (without radiographic evidence of bone metastases on complete skeletal survey).

Our approach – surgery to the exclusion of radiation and chemotherapy, except as outlined above – seems to be vindicated in all stages except Stage III[6]. Here it becomes evident that radiation prolongs the survival of Stage III patients. In the light of present knowledge we believe that the greater the bulk of the tumor left behind, the more difficult the cure. In Stage III, tumors cross the midline and hence are difficult to resect because they cannot be reached, as in the mediastinum, or they surround a vital structure such as the celiac axis (Table II). The staging scheme supports the earlier concept of better prognosis under one year, but the anatomic site has lost its prognostic importance: it is the stage, not the site, which determines survival. Staging does not differentiate between degrees of malignant histology.

The respective roles of surgery and radiation are further delineated by comparing our series with 100 patients in co-operative Group A[1]. Our patients were treated according to the precepts already discussed: those in Group A all had postoperative radiation to the tumor bed or residual tumor, as well as chemotherapy. In comparing our series with those of Group A, it is clear that although there are no statistically significant differences, the survival of our patients without radiation and chemotherapy was at least as good as those in Group A. For example, the co-operative group reported a survival of 60% in Stage II and 13% in Stage III while our figures were 80% and 11% respectively[6].

TABLE II

134 Neuroblastomas: Children's Hospital of Philadelphia

	Stage						
Age (Yr.)	I	II	III	IV	IV^S	Total	Per Cent
<1	8/9	10/11	2/4	2/13	8/8	30/45	67
<2	3/4	2/4	2/3	0/17	–	7/28	25
2+	1/1	2/5	3/9	1/45	1/1	8/61	13
Total (per cent)	86	70	44	4	100		34

With respect to the influence of chemotherapy, 43% of the irradiated patients in the co-operative group survived when given chemotherapy, whereas 77% of the irradiated patients in the Children's Hospital of Philadelphia survived without chemotherapy. Although these series are small, it seems obvious that the addition of chemotherapy does not improve survival.

All our children in Stage IV^S have survived; few of them received radiation, and chemotherapy has been used only recently. In the co-operative group, deaths of two children in Stage IV^S were due to the effects of these modes of therapy.

RHABDOMYOSARCOMA

Rhabdomyosarcoma is the most common soft-tissue sarcoma in children. The existence of three, if not four, histological varieties of this tumor suggests differing prognoses. The traditional teaching that rhabdomyosarcomas are not radiosensitive is false, and a variety of chemotherapeutic agents, alone or in combination, are apparently effective against some forms of this tumor.

Our own experience is limited to 40 patients, 33 of whom were treated more than two years ago. The survival rate in these 33 patients is 38%[7]. We have compared our results with three other series, those of the Children's Hospital of Pittsburgh[8], the Children's Hospital of Columbus, Ohio[9], and the Mayo Clinic[10]. The survival rate in these combined series was 29%.

The staging scheme for rhabdomyosarcoma helps in making these comparisons: Stage I lesions are those tumors localized to the primary site of the tumor. Stage II lesions are those with a local or regional extension. The Pittsburgh group have further subdivided Stage II lesions into subgroups based upon resectability and non-resectability of the tumor. Stage III lesions are those that presented with known distant metastases.

Patients under one year of age with rhabdomyosarcoma do poorly as contrasted with those with neuroblastoma or Wilms' tumor. The site of the lesion had some relationship to survival, the extremities having the best and the pelvis the poorest prognosis.

Aggressive, non-mutilative surgery combined with radiation and chemotherapy seems to be responsible for improved results and should be vigorously pursued.

SUMMARY

Neuroblastomas localized to the organ of origin (Stage I) are usually resectable and the survival rate in our hands is 86%. When neuroblastomas extend beyond the organ of origin but do not cross the midline (Stage II), excision of the major portion of the tumor results in a 70% survival. Radiation therapy does not improve the results in Stages I and II. In Stage III tumors, the neuroblastoma has spread across the midline and partial resection followed by radiation therapy gives a better survival than partial resection alone. The presence of bone metastasis in neuroblastoma is almost universally fatal. A special group of patients with neuroblastoma who have metastasis to the liver, skin, or bone marrow (or any combination thereof) seems to do well with excision of the primary tumor (where possible) but require no adjunctive therapy.

In the management of rhabdomyosarcoma, surgical excision still remains the primary weapon. Because the rhabdomyosarcoma is sensitive to radiation therapy and to a variety of chemotherapeutic agents, surgical procedures should be extirpative but should avoid amputation where possible. The aggressive use of radiotherapy and chemotherapy has produced better survival rates than were previously reported with surgery alone.

REFERENCES

1 EVANS, A. E., D'ANGIO, G. J. and RANDOLPH, J.: A proposed staging for children with neuroblastoma. *Cancer,* **27:** 374, 1971.

2 KOOP, C. E. and HERNANDEZ, J. R.: Neuroblastoma: Experience with 100 cases in children. *Surgery,* **56:** 726, 1964.

3 KOOP, C. E., HOPE, J. W. and ABIR, E.: Management of nephroblastoma (Wilms' tumor) and abdominal neuroblastoma. *CA,* **14:** 178, 1964.

4 KOOP, C. E., KIESEWETTER, W. B. and HORN, R. C.: Neuroblastoma in childhood: An evaluation of surgical management. *Pediatrics,* **16:** 625, 1955.

5 KOOP, C. E., KIESEWETTER, W. B. and HORN, R. C.: Neuroblastoma in childhood. *Surgery,* **38:** 272, 1955.

6 KOOP, C. E. and JOHNSON, D. G.: Neuroblastoma: An assessment of therapy in reference to staging. *J Pediatr Surg,* **6:** 595, 1971.

7 KOOP, C. E. and TEWARSON, I. P.: Rhabdomyosarcoma of the head and neck in children. *Ann Surg,* **160:** 95, 1964.

8 EHRLICH, F. E., HAAS, J. E. and KIESEWETTER, W. B.: Rhabdomyosarcoma in infants and children: Factors affecting long-term survival. *J Pediatr Surg,* **6:** 571, 1971.

9 GROSFELD, J. L., CLATWORTHY, H. W., Jr. and NEWTON, W. A., Jr.: Combined therapy in childhood rhabdomyosarcomas: An analysis of 42 cases. *J Pediatr Surg,* **4:** 637, 1969.

10 MAHOUR, R. C., SOULE, E. H., MILLS, S. D. and LYNN, H. B.: Rhabdomyosarcoma in infants and children: A clinicopathological study of 75 cases. *J Pediatr Surg,* **2:** 402, 1967.

PANEL ON RHABDOMYOSARCOMA AND NEUROBLASTOMA

Moderator: C. A. STEPHENS*
Panelists: G. J. D'ANGIO**, J. M. M. DARTE†, C. E. KOOP‡, O. SCHWEISGUTH‡, J. R. WILBUR††, and P. B. DENT‡‡

Dr. Stephens: Would the panel discuss more fully the treatment of the patient with Stage IV^S neuroblastoma? This infant presents with a huge liver full of secondary tumor (the primary may or may not be obvious) and there is usually no other obvious metastatic disease.

Dr. Schweisguth: While some have advocated supportive treatment only or vitamin B12 alone in infants with Stage IV^S neuroblastoma, we have had only one child survive with supportive care only. I think it is highly unusual for these infants to survive without treatment, and that at least some treatment is necessary to initiate tumor regression. The infant usually presents with a rapidly enlarging liver. At this time, the weight gain, which can be as much as 100-200 grams a day, is represented by an increase in weight of the liver. We have lost some infants, as I mentioned, in the first few days in hospital because the enormous growth of the liver was just too much for the infant and it died. To help them, we rely on biochemistry for diagnosis and do not do an initial laparotomy in these small infants. We treat them initially with irradiation, using 1000 rads given through two lateral fields, thus protecting the kidney. This dose is usually adequate to initiate regression of the tumor. We watch them closely and sometimes use chemotherapy in addition, depending on their progress and hematological status. Sometimes these infants with large livers have thrombocytopenia – I do not know why – and this may be important because, in my opinion, it complicates the use of chemotherapy. We wait until the liver and the VMA are normal or nearly so and then do a laparotomy and remove the primary tumor. At the time of laparotomy one finds only residual fibrosis in the liver. We have never found a single ganglioneuroma cell in the liver, so we think the neuroblastoma cells are destroyed and do not mature in the liver. At the primary site, it is usually still possible to recognize neuroblastoma histologically. We believe the primary tumor has to be removed but then, if the clinical situation is

*The Hospital for Sick Children, Toronto.
**Memorial Hospital for Cancer and Allied Diseases, New York.
†Charles A. Janeway Child Health Centre, St. John's, Newfoundland.
‡The Children's Hospital of Philadelphia, Philadelphia, Pa., U.S.A.
‡Institut Gustave-Roussy, Villejuif, France.
††The Children's Hospital at Stanford, Palo Alto, Calif., U.S.A.
‡‡Department of Pediatrics, McMaster University, Hamilton.

satisfactory, we do nothing else. We use initial irradiation, occasionally a few months of chemotherapy and then surgical excision of the primary. That is all. What do you do, Dr. Koop?

Dr. Koop: What Dr. Schweisguth has said is logical and I would not object to her management. I do not do it that way. I would go after the primary initially and excise it, if possible. I would not add further specific treatment unless the subsequent progress was unsatisfactory. When we have had occasion to take a second look in these infants, we have never found any ganglioneuroma in the liver nor have we been able to find any ganglioneuroma cells in the subcutaneous nodules, even though these may be present initially.

Dr. Stephens: Have you been faced with a situation where you did not know where the primary was?

Dr. Koop: I have been faced with a situation where I could not find the primary and, therefore, have not gone after it.

Dr. Stephens: You would irradiate that child?

Dr. Koop: No, no irradiation at all! And all alive, don't forget that!

Dr. D'Angio: The important thing here, quite obviously, is that we do not really understand Stage IV^S. I agree wholeheartedly that they tend to be overtreated rather than the opposite. A particular problem relates to the extent of bone-marrow involvement, and whether these infants should continue to be included in the IV^S category. On the one hand, one may see actual rosettes in the bone marrow and, on the other, only sheets of lymphoblast-like cells that Audrey Evans has described so well, and which perhaps are immunoblasts rather than tumor cells. If the infant has rosettes in the bone marrow, the decision whether an infant is in the IV^S constellation rather than Stage IV with skeletal involvement, depends on the excellence of the radiographs and the skill of the radiologist in reading the films. In these patients at least, one might consider using a pulse of chemotherapy of a kind that does not give the marked toxicity of maintained cyclic agents.

Looking back on the history of neuroblastoma, one finds that some of these infants have been given nitrogen mustard with good effect. At the present time, perhaps one should use only nitrogen mustard as a single unmaintained agent rather than vincristine and cytoxan in a maintained cyclic fashion, as has been popular more recently.

Dr. Schweisguth: I do not believe that the toxicity of vincristine and cytoxan is very great. I would prefer not to use nitrogen mustard. Of our 38 infants with Stage IV^S disease, many had evidence of bone marrow dissemination at the time of diagnosis. We have lost five of these later with gross metastatic bone disease. We have no way of telling which patient will go on to gross bone disease. We, therefore, prefer to treat with chemotherapy those with bone marrow involvement. As with Wilms' tumor, we may be treating some of them unnecessarily.

Dr. Darte: We are getting to the core of the problem in trying to clarify the nature of bone marrow metastasis. We have always been very reluctant to call a bone marrow positive without very clear evidence of disseminated tumor cells. However, when in doubt we have usually treated the patient systemically. Nowadays, we culture bone marrow and have been getting very good growth of neuroblastoma. We find this a more sensitive method of detecting neuroblastoma seeding in the bone marrow than looking at slides where there are always cells which you are never quite sure of. It takes only 48-72 hours to get a reading on a neuroblastoma marrow aspirate in culture. Likewise, in a suspicious lymph node, we take one-half and culture it and believe the results are more definite than the usual morphological characteristics. I do not have good results in children with bone marrow metastases, most of these die within a few months with obvious radiological changes. Perhaps this is because we only classify, as involved, those marrows about which we are absolutely certain.

Dr. Stephens: Do you believe the prognosis is worse for a child who has radiological evidence of bone involvement, as opposed to one with just bone marrow evidence or cultural evidence of tumor cells?

Dr. Darte: I cannot answer the question about cultural characteristics yet. We have been doing this for about a year and we do not have that many cases. There seems to be a good correlation between positive cultures and later gross evidence of bone involvement.

Dr. Stephens. A question for Dr. Koop. Should the child who has bone marrow involvement, but who is responding to treatment, have his primary removed?

Dr. Koop: It has been my practice to do so but I cannot defend it on scientific grounds. It just seems logical and, being a surgeon, if I have a tumor that I can take out, I do not leave it there. Whether or not the removal of the primary affects the metastasis, I do not know. I would not jeopardize the child's life to do so, nor would I do it in an extemely sick child but, given a child who is on the mend and who is going up instead of down and has a primary that I can get out, I will take it out.

Dr. Stephens: If taking it out would jeopardize life, you probably would not?

Dr. Koop: No!

Dr. Schweisguth: And how many successes have you had in children with metastases after taking out the primary?

Dr. Koop: If gross bone metastasis were present, we have had no successes, but 50% of our surviving patients had soft-tissue metastases, proven histologically.

Dr. Stephens: In those cases where you did a partial dissection, did you ever encounter uncontrolled bleeding?

Dr. Koop: No, I never did. I have got into situations where I regretted that I had gone that far. As I get older, I get a lot more cautious. I do make a very small incision and test the vascularity of the tumor. I do not make sweeping incisions and just go after that big thing with a spoon. I do it very gently and if it starts to work I continue. If it does not, I beat a hasty and judicious retreat.

Dr. Stephens: We have had two children die on the table while attempting partial resection, after starting out to do total resection, because of uncontrolled bleeding.

I have a question now asking for more information on some of the newer chemotherapeutic agents in rhabdomyosarcoma such as Adriamycin. Would anyone like to comment?

Dr. Wilbur: I would be glad to answer that for a number of reasons. It has been interesting to sit and hear the radiotherapists say how great radiotherapy is, and the surgeon say how great surgery is, and yet there has not been an adequate discussion of chemotherapy, which is the best therapy for rhabdomyosarcoma. This is not to exclude irradiation therapy and surgery but rather to indicate that chemotherapy is now playing a major role in treatment. I can best illustrate this by just giving one portion of our results at the M. D. Anderson Hospital in Houston. Dr. Koop mentioned a 23% survival in head and neck rhabdomyosarcoma. In a recent review of our patients with inoperable rhabdomyosarcoma of the nasopharynx and oropharynx, nine of 11 patients are surviving from two to five years after treatment with irradiation and combination chemotherapy using vincristine, actinomycin-D and cyclophosphamide. In this type of tumor, which in the past has almost been uniformly fatal, at least two-thirds are now surviving over prolonged periods. All nine of these have completed two years of chemotherapy and are now off all drugs. The child with the longest survival has been off chemotherapy for three years. No doubt some of these children will recur at some time in the future but perhaps some will not.

We used vincristine, actinomycin-D and cyclophosphamide in combination initially, but Adriamycin is an effective agent, which will produce significant regression of disease in a high proportion of patients. Its major limitation is cardiotoxicity, which will occur above a certain cumulative dose. We use 500 milligrams per square metre as the upper limit but this upper limit may have to be reduced further. It is a significant medication and may well have a place in combination therapy together with vincristine, actinomycin-D and cyclophosphamide.

Dr. Stephens: In a patient with rhabdomyosarcoma of an extremity where there is a reasonable chance of getting a complete surgical excision, would you treat with chemotherapy or with surgery?

Dr. Wilbur: I was not implying that surgery had no role. If one can remove a tumor without causing severe distress to the patient, either in terms of morbidity or mortality or significant disfigurement, surgery is the first choice of therapy. However, treatment usually cannot stop at that point because the common cause of death in rhabdomyosarcoma is the distant spread of disease. If using chemotherapy you can eradicate occult metastatic disease, which cannot be demonstrated at the time of initial treatment, survival rates will be higher.

Dr. Koop: Lest the audience misinterpret what I had to say about surgery and rhabdomyosarcoma, as Dr. Wilbur perhaps did, let me say that I showed those patients with head and neck lesions to imply strongly that surgery was ineffective, in that I left tumor behind, but that the patients are alive and well because of chemotherapy.

Dr. Stephens: Following a local surgical incision, when a tumor was known to be left behind, would you use irradiation and chemotherapy, or chemotherapy alone?

Dr. Koop: After a local surgical procedure, and whether or not I was certain that there was tumor left behind, I would give chemotherapy postoperatively without irradiation.

Dr. D'Angio. After a local surgical procedure with no microscopic residual disease, I believe postoperative irradiation is indicated.

May I ask Dr. Wilbur a question? What are the results of chemotherapy in Stage IV?

Dr. Wilbur: In our patients with metastatic disease to distant sites in a group treated since 1967, four of eight are alive with no evidence of disease more than two years after their treatment.

Dr. Stephens: I can answer a question that was directed to Dr. Ein who is not here. Will you explain Wilms' tumor of the liver? Do these children have primary Wilms' tumor in the liver?

The answer to that is no! These were secondary Wilms' tumors metastatic in liver.

Question: Are blocking antibodies tumor specific?

Dr. Dent: To the best of our knowledge, in both experimental animal and clinical situations, serum blocking factors are tumor-specific. This observation has been used to prove the specificity of lymphocyte cytotoxicity reactions *in vitro.* When allogeneic mixtures of tumor cells and lymphocytes are cultured together *in vitro,* the lymphocytes will eventually attack and destroy the tumor cells. Blocking antibody directed against the tumor-specific antigens will not prevent this reaction, which is dependent upon histocompatability differences between the lymphocytes and target cells. It will, however, block any tumor-specific cytotoxic reactions.

Dr. Sinks: In relation to Dr. Dent's presentation, I would like to comment on carcinoembryonic antigen which may become a valuable tool in the management of neuroblastoma. Last spring, Dr. Wang of our department, presented data to show that carcinoembryonic antigen, which was regarded as specific for colonic malignancy at one time is, in fact, nonspecific. In a study of approximately 17 children with neuroblastoma, we found that carcinoembroyonic antigen titres were elevated above normal when the disease was active. When these children were treated successfully and all clinical evidence of the disease was eradicated, the carcinoembryonic antigen titre fell below normal. In one instance, it remained positive and anticipated the clinical recurrence of disease by at least four weeks. The only false-positive was in a 17-year-old girl who, during infancy, had received irradiation for a neuroblastoma, metastatic to the liver. At the time of the test she was pregnant. Estimates of carcinoembryonic antigen titres may prove to be a better quantitative assessment of tumor activity than catacholamine excretion, although it is much too early to be definite about this.

Question: Would you proceed to a radical surgical excision of a rhabdomyosarcoma on the basis of a frozen section alone?

Dr. Koop: It is hard to find a pathologist willing to do this, at least in our community. I cannot recall any time in the past seven years when we have done this but it has been done and I know of no errors.

Dr. Stephens: One more question. Is the site of neuroblastoma not of value in prognosis, for example, neck, groin or pelvis?

Dr. Koop: It is of some value but I think the reason these sites are associated with a good prognosis is that a greater proportion of these tumors are Stage I. The concept that certain sites are associated with a better prognosis is valid. However, it is better to cover prognosis within a general staging system rather than any anatomical device.

Dr. D'Angio: I would like to emphasize what Dr. Koop said. We have analyzed this and confirmed that it is the stage that matters. For example, Stage III in the thorax has a bad prognosis. It is the stage that counts.

Dr. Schweisguth: I would like to comment on rhabdomyosarcoma. I think our main difficulty has been to control this disease at the primary site, and it is only when we are able to do this that control of remote disease becomes relevant. We have treated a number of children with localized disease by means of interstitial implantation. In patients suitable for this treatment we have had very good results. In particular, in two children who had vaginal rhabdomyosarcoma of the botryoid type, the disease has been controlled by interstitial irradiation. Radical surgery, which in this situation may mean excision of the bladder and/or rectum, has been avoided. One of these girls was treated at age 11 and is now well three years later. She is menstruating normally and her only morbidity is a moderate vaginal stenosis.

Dr. D'Angio: I disagree with Dr. Schweisguth, to some extent, when she says that no progress had been made in relation to neuroblastoma. Not only are there some promising leads but we are beginning to understand this tumor better. Therapeutically, however, we have not been able to make much improvement in the survival rate. Part of this may be because a proportion of these children respond very poorly to chemotherapy. It is worth recalling here that, as Dr. Freireich pointed out, unless you have a better than 50% response rate to any form of therapy you are not going to see any difference in median survival because 50% die early. The median survival is the same but the two survival curves may still plateau at different levels. What we really need is a method of getting an early indication of whether the patient is responding to any particular therapy. We could then be particularly energetic in our treatment of this more favorable group, while continuing to search for agents that are effective in a higher proportion of patients.

Dr. Stephens: A question for Dr. D'Angio. In Stages I and II neuroblastoma, do you use any form of treatment other than surgery?

Dr. D'Angio: For Stage I tumors, I now believe that surgery alone is adequate. Survival rates are good but there are failures. Most of these result from distant disease. In Stage II, Dr. Koop's data again shows no difference between irradiated and nonirradiated groups even when the surgical excision is known to be incomplete. For this reason, I think at present we should not give postoperative irradiation. However, the numbers in Stage II from the Children's Hospital in Philadelphia are small so that it is difficult to be sure. Dr. Koop has been a pioneer in this whole field and I am much indebted to him for his demonstration of the nature of this tumor. In Stage III, there is no doubt that further treatment has to be given.

Dr. Shandling: Does Dr. D'Angio agree with the recommendation to go after a small primary, say in Stage IV^S?

Dr. D'Angio: Yes, I think so, but let me say once again, it depends very much on who the surgeon is. When Dr. Koop says that he can go after a primary in an abdomen distended by a grossly enlarged metastatic liver, that is one thing; but for the casual surgeon who does not have all the full back-up or experience, that is another. Again, it depends on the experience of the individual institution. When the primary is left in, the risk is that it may dedifferentiate back to neuroblastoma, but this is a rare event, so you take relative risks, it seems to me. If the operation is simple and the tumor small, on balance, I would favor the procedure. However, in many hospitals it may be that the risk of attempting surgery is greater than that with a conservative approach. I realize that that is an indefinite answer. I do not think you have to take the primary out in order to get survival.

Dr. Darte: I think Dr. Shandling is aware that we do not take out the primary usually in Stage IV^S disease. I do not think our survival rate is different and I have never seen a late relapse from primary recurrence.

Dr. Schweisguth: We remove the primary after initial control of the liver lesion because we had one child recur at the primary site five years after diagnosis.

Dr. D'Angio: But that is very rare. There is perhaps a 2% chance that this may happen but is the surgical mortality less than that?

Dr. Schweisguth: Surgical removal of the primary after the liver has reverted to normal is usually straightforward. If the tumor is in the celiac region, it is usually inoperable and we do not try. But, in most cases, the tumor is suprarenal and you just find a small adrenal gland with a normal cortex but with a sclerotic medulla with a few residual neuroblastoma cells.

Dr. Stephens: I agree to some extent with Dr. Koop that, in some of these children with huge livers from secondary involvement, it may not be terribly difficult to remove the primary before irradiation.

Dr. Schweisguth: I do not see the value of doing that.

Dr. Koop: You are not a surgeon!

Dr. Sonley: There is very much more tumor in the enlarged liver. How do you explain the fact that the liver can be controlled but the primary may not be?

Dr. Schweisguth: I do not explain it – if I could, they would give me the Nobel Prize!

Dr. Sonley: All the major centres around the world have about the same results, so it would appear that it does not matter which of several treatment methods you use.

PANEL ON PSYCHIATRIC PROBLEMS IN THE MANAGEMENT OF CHILDREN WITH MALIGNANCY

Moderator: M. J. SONLEY*
Panelists: E. H. PAKES**, J. KIKUCHI†, and J. M. M. DARTE‡

(Dr. Pakes, a psychiatrist at the Hospital for Sick Children, who is particularly interested in children with leukemia, had recently been appointed Consultant to the Children's Ward of Princess Margaret Hospital; Miss June Kikuchi, clinical nurse, the Hospital for Sick Children, works solely with children with leukemia and their families; and Dr. John Darte, Professor of Pediatrics at Memorial University, Newfoundland, has had a long experience in caring for children with malignancy.)

Rather than have the panel describe what they believed the patients and their parents felt, two videotapes were shown in which the parents and one of the patients express their own views.

The first tape showed a discussion between Miss Kikuchi and a 15-year-old boy with acute leukemia that had been diagnosed one year previously. He said he was glad he had been told the diagnosis because he could discuss his problems and concerns more meaningfully with his parents, friends and the doctors. He described how the disease and its medications had seriously curtailed his sports activities and his social life. He felt that the doctors and nurses didn't talk enough about the disease to him and he wanted to know more about the side effects of drugs at the time they were given, rather than after the effects had appeared. He wanted to speak to other children with the same diagnosis and thought they might help each other by discussing how to deal with the problems associated with their disease, and with their parents' concern about their illness.

The second videotape showed a discussion between four sets of parents and Dr. Pakes. The children of two sets of parents had recently died. The parents were concerned about how the diagnosis was revealed to them. They thought that they should not be told over the phone or in the hallway of the hospital, which happened to two of them. Both parents should be present, and sitting down and comfortable. They urged the doctor to make himself familiar with the current prognosis so as not to give the parents a too-gloomy prognosis unnecessarily. Some revealed their anger that their child had developed cancer.

*The Princess Margaret Hospital, Toronto.
**The Hospital for Sick Children, Toronto.
†The Hospital for Sick Children, Toronto.
‡Charles A. Janeway Child Health Centre, St. John's, Newfoundland.

They were concerned about whether the child should be told his diagnosis and his prognosis. They discussed the effect of the illness on the other siblings and on their marriage, and their attempts to prepare themselves for the death long before it happens. They felt that, when all hope was gone and when the doctors were maintaining life for only a few days, they should be told that there was no hope and given some idea of when he might die. They did not want their child to suffer unnecessarily to prolong his life for a few days. They stressed their need to be kept informed and their desire to have a room on the ward where they could have a few minutes to themselves during the day away from their own and other children. They felt that they, as well as their children, were "patients" and they wished to be considered as individuals with needs and wants of their own.

During the question period, a member of the audience asked whether most of the stress in the "psychiatric management" is on preparing the patient and parents for the death of the child, or whether the parents of children who had never had a relapse of their disease weren't treated more optimistically. The panel agreed that the parents were given a realistic prognosis but that, initially, an optimistic outlook was stressed. Emphasis was placed on the research being done in the disease, the recent improvements in therapy and the possibility that their child could survive. However, after the first or second relapse, the parents' initial optimism is replaced by concern about the eventual demise of the child, and the staff then attempt to help the parents deal with this through discussion with the doctors, nurses and by parent discussion groups, in which they share their feelings and help each other.

A member of the audience suggested that not only the parents needed treatment, but that the residents, nurses and doctors looking after the children had to come to terms with their own views about death. Dr. Pakes pointed out that the professional staff also has to go through the mourning process, and that they gain support from each other. This often happens at ward rounds and at meetings similar to this one. Not only the parents, but also the professional staff benefit from group discussions.

Someone asked whether children who know their diagnoses and are about to die are told that they are dying, and if so how. The panel felt that one should not deny an imminent death if the patient mentions it, and that one should allow the patient to express his feelings about it freely. The doctor should assure him that he is not going to be left alone; that he is not going to be abandoned just because he is no longer receiving active therapy. It is tempting for the professional staff to look in the door of a dying patient and discover that the patient is sleeping or apparently busy and decide to pass the room quickly, so as not to have to face him. The dying patient should be visited at least as frequently as when there was hope for the future. The young patient should be reassured about things which might be worrying them, for example that a leg would not be amputated or that some of the frightening things they had seen happen to other patients should not happen to them, and that they will have adequate analgesia for pain.

Finally, someone asked why the whole family could not be included in the discussions about the illness rather than having only parent groups or discussions with the patients themselves. The panel agreed that the siblings also have problems in dealing with their feelings about the illness and that this could be handled effectively in group therapy, and subsequent intrapersonal problems might be prevented.

THE VALUE OF LAPAROTOMY IN THE STAGING OF HODGKIN'S DISEASE IN CHILDREN

C. A. STEPHENS, M.D., F.R.C.S.(C)*

In most children with Hodgkin's disease, spleen and liver scans, intravenous pyelography, inferior vena cavagrams, gastrointestinal series and barium enema studies have failed to delineate the extent of subdiaphragmatic lymph-node or organ involvement. Pedal lymphangiograms have been of some value in detecting involved retroperitoneal lymph nodes, but this examination does not demonstrate nodes in the region of the celiac axis. Definitely positive lymphangiograms are very helpful, but negative examinations cannot be relied upon. Because of this, since 1968, 25 children with histologically-proven Hodgkin's disease have been submitted to laparotomy to determine the extent of abdominal visceral and retroperitoneal gland involvement.

These 25 children ranged in age from three years to 17 years; 75% were over 10 years of age. Sixteen had radiological evidence of mediastinal lymph-node involvement; in the other nine, the mediastinal glands appeared to be free of disease radiologically. The subdiaphragmatic involvement in these two groups of patients, however, were very similar. Sixty-two per cent of the children with mediastinal disease had involvement below the diaphragm and 55% of those without evidence of mediastinal involvement had disease below the diaphragm – involving either retroperitoneal glands or spleen, or both.

Pedal lymphangiography, which had been done in 24 patients before operation, was reported positive for retroperitoneal lymph-node involvement in seven, and normal in 17. At laparotomy, histological examination of retroperitoneal lymph-node biopsies confirmed that disease was present in six of the seven reported as positive by lymphangiography. (The seventh had had preoperative abdominal radiation.) It also revealed that, of the 17 whose lymphangiograms were reported as normal, five had definite retroperitoneal or abdominal visceral disease and several pathologists reviewing the sections could not agree on two others. This experience supports the contention that positive lymphangiograms are very helpful but negative ones are not reliable.

In summary, of the 25 children with Hodgkin's disease undergoing laparotomy, 16 had disease below the diaphragm (in two more there was a difference of pathological opinion). This involvement was suspected in six on the basis of preoperative lymphangiograms, and in one on the basis of marked splenomegaly with hypersplenism. Spleen and retroperitoneal glands were involved in 10 children, the spleen alone in three, and the retroperitoneal glands

*Division of General Surgery, The Hospital for Sick Children, Toronto.

alone in three (± 2 with pathological dispute). The gross appearance of the spleen, in most cases, did not provide an accurate indication of its involvement.

Five children had postoperative complications. Three had an adhesive small bowel obstruction; two recovered on conservative treatment, one required surgical treatment. One child developed pneumonia postoperatively which responded promptly to antibiotic therapy. One child developed a viral encephalitis while receiving radiotherapy and chemotherapy in the postoperative period. This child finally died of Hodgkin's disease.

If the premise is valid that Hodgkin's disease is curable if all involved areas are adequately treated, laparotomy appears to have a place as a staging tool. In addition, some surgeons recommend biopsies of the iliac crest and sternum to rule out bone marrow involvement, and others recommend routine biopsy of the periportal and mesenteric lymph nodes. In this series, mesenteric nodes were biopsied only if they appeared abnormal on gross examination. None of these biopsies were positive. At the time of laparotomy, in the female patient, the ovaries should be fixed and marked with a radiopaque clip outside the field of possible abdominal radiation.

NON-HODGKIN'S LYMPHOMA IN CHILDREN

JORDAN R. WILBUR, M.D.*, MARTIN MOTT, M.B., M.R.C.P.**,
MARGARET SULLIVAN, M.D.†, and W. W. SUTOW, M.D.‡

Non-Hodgkin's lymphoma (lymphosarcoma) in childhood is a complex topic which cannot be completely discussed in a short presentation. The following summary is based on a review of children treated in the last five years at the University of Texas M. D. Anderson Hospital and Tumor Institute in Houston, Texas. Before presenting this information it is important to review the problems and limitations encountered in any attempt to compare one institution's data concerning the treatment of non-Hodgkin's lymphoma in children with that of any other institution.

A primary problem is to achieve agreement among pathologists, hematologists and oncologists as to exactly which diseases we are talking about. The nomenclature is variable and seems to be continually changing. What one pathologist diagnoses as a diffuse, poorly differentiated lymphoblastic lymphoma, another may label an undifferentiated lymphosarcoma. Other names including reticulum cell sarcoma, poorly differentiated lymphosarcoma or extramedullary leukemia are also used. Secondly, lymphomas in children are frequently compared with those occurring in adults. Most of the non-Hodgkin's lymphomas in children are diffuse in contrast with the frequently nodular lymphomas in adults. The pattern and frequency of spread of the disease to other sites varies between adults and children. In general, the disease more commonly spreads in children. Hence we must determine at what age the lymphoma acts like the tumor of childhood rather than that of the adult. The teenager with lymphoma generally has a pattern of spread similar to that of younger children.

Since the incidence of non-Hodgkin's lymphoma in childhood is relatively low, few institutions see a sufficiently large number of patients over a relatively short time to allow any statistically significant evaluation of treatment or results. Thus. series of patients from individual institutions may cover a span of many years. This presents additional problems. The first is that of staging. How

---

*Director, Children's Oncology Unit, Children's Hospital, Stanford, Palo Alto, California. (Formerly, Head, Department of Pediatrics, University of Texas M.D. Anderson Hospital, Houston, Texas.)

**Project Investigator, Department of Pediatrics, University of Texas M. D. Anderson Hospital, Houston, Texas. (Formerly, Department of Pediatrics, University of Bristol, Bristol, England.)

†Associate Professor of Pediatrics, University of Texas M. D. Anderson Hospital, Houston, Texas.

‡Professor of Pediatrics, University of Texas M. D. Anderson Hospital, Houston, Texas.

complete was the staging which determined the extent of the disease? Was lymphangiography included? Was a staging laparotomy done? Was a bone marrow biopsy done or simply a bone marrow aspiration? Another problem with evaluating patients over an extended time span is that the therapy has changed greatly. Recent changes include improved chemotherapy and radiation therapy. Improvements in supportive therapy include platelet transfusions and better antibiotics. This improved treatment of complications has permitted more intensive therapy. Due to these improvements, we cannot use length of survival over a short period as a meaningful measure when comparing one institution's earlier results with treatment in recent years.

The location and specific type of disease also influences results. The location of the primary appears to be a significant factor in predicting the expected course of the disease. A major question here is whether or not the disease will progress to a "leukemic transformation". For example, a primary in the mediastinum is much more frequently associated with leukemic transformation than one located in the abdomen[1]. Here again we must classify leukemic transformation. Does this represent the infiltration of the bone marrow by malignant cells or the appearance of malignant cells in the circulating blood? How frequently does the disease spread to the central nervous system? This last is an important question, both in terms of therapeutic results, and the inclusion of prophylactic therapy to the central nervous system. However, in studying either leukemic transformation or central-nervous-system spread, the data must be evaluated, considering whether the patients survived long enough to develop these secondary changes.

Other factors must also be considered. Has the evaluated group been specially selected in any way? For example, is the group limited to patients seen by radiotherapists, i.e., does it not include those who have already developed leukemic transformation? Are the patients those seen in a referral centre, who represent only those well enough to qualify for studies there and well enough to travel to get there? On the other hand, do they represent mainly patients who have progressive disease and are being sent to a centre for more experimental therapy because their disease is progressing? Are patients who have had previous therapy included in the evaluation? Has the length of time from first symptomatology to diagnosis been considered in evaluating response to therapy and survival time? All of these variables must be considered in evaluating response to therapy.

To simplify the classification of non-Hodgkin's lymphoma in children at M. D. Anderson Hospital, they are grouped into three classifications: differentiated lymphoma, Burkitt's type; undifferentiated lymphoma, non-Burkitt's type; and histiocytic lymphoma[2]. Although the undifferentiated lymphoma of the American Burkitt's type can be differentiated from the non-Burkitt's type by pathologic criteria, the clinical progression of disease and response to therapy are frequently similar. Therefore, in considering therapy of non-Hodgkin's lymphoma in children, we make a clear distinction only between histiocytic lymphoma and the undifferentiated lymphomas.

All of these limitations should be kept in mind when evaluating the children with non-Hodgkin's lymphoma treated during the period 1968 to 1972 at the University of Texas M. D. Anderson Hospital. To minimize some of the variables previously noted, this report will concentrate on patients with histiocytic lymphoma – a type which most pathologists agree upon and in which the general prognosis has been uniformly poor. The percentage of long-term survivors regardless of pathologic type varies between 10 and 30% and generally is not satisfactory[3-7]. The survival rate in histiocytic lymphoma has been even more dismal. At M. D. Anderson Hospital before 1968, all eight children with histiocytic lymphoma died within one year.

However, more intensive combination chemotherapy given in conjunction with radiation therapy and with more intensive and improved supportive therapy, may allow increasing numbers of children with non-Hodgkin's lymphoma not only to survive longer but to recover totally.

Of the 12 children with histiocytic lymphoma treated between 1968 and 1971, six are still alive, four without evidence of disease since their initial program. This group of patients will be reviewed year by year.

In 1968, four patients with histiocytic lymphoma of childhood were diagnosed. With standard cyclophosphamide-vincristine-prednisone therapy, all four died in an average time of six months; one survived as long as one year. In 1969, two children with histiocytic lymphoma were treated on a new program which still included prednisone and vincristine but with very intensive cyclophosphamide therapy – a dose of 15 mg./kg./day for up to 10 days. The course of therapy was interrupted if the total granulocyte count dropped below 1000. Intensive radiation therapy was also given to the local area of disease. Both of these patients had Stage I disease. They are continuing to do well now three years after completion of their therapy. Of the two patients with histiocytic lymphoma treated in 1970, both died within less than six months, one a failure on the same intensive cyclophosphamide program. The other patient had had a significant amount of previous radiation therapy and could not tolerate an intensive chemotherapy program.

In 1971, doxorubicin (Adriamycin) was added to the therapeutic program. The initial treatment is indicated in Fig. 1. Following completion of the Adriamycin therapy, which was limited owing to potential cardiac toxicity, the program was changed to intensive cyclophosphamide therapy. The four patients treated in 1971, who included one each in Stages I, II, III and IV, are all still alive at this time. The two with Stages III and IV disease have had recurrences and, although some control has been achieved, they are not expected to live long. The other two continue to do well at this time without evidence of recurrent disease. In addition to chemotherapy, they have received intensive radiation therapy to the involved lymph nodes.

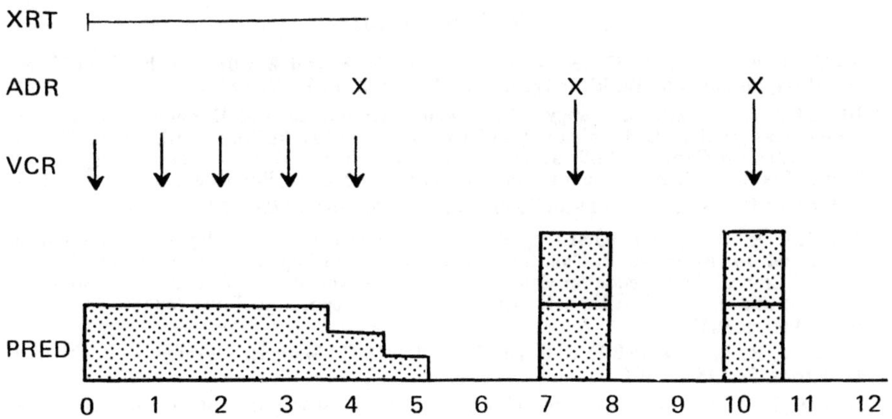

Doses

VCR =	**Vincristine**	2 mg./m^2 IV (max. 2 mg.)
PRED =	**Prednisone**	60 mg./m^2/d (max. 60 mg.) for 4 weeks; Beginning week 7, 120 mg./m^2/d (max. 120 mg.) for 5 days
ADR =	**Adriamycin**	60 mg./m^2 single IV dose – q 3 weeks x 8 doses
XRT =	**Radiotherapy**	

Fig. 1. VAP (vincristine-Adriamycin-prednisone) therapy for histiocytic lymphoma in children.

Although the numbers are small and the time relatively short, these results represent a significant improvement over the results achieved before 1968 when no patient with histiocytic lymphoma in childhood treated at M. D. Anderson Hospital survived for one year.

In 1971, we treated four children with non-Burkitt's lymphoma or undifferentiated lymphoma of childhood. Only one of the four has died and the other three are doing well without evidence of recurrent disease at 12, 12 and 22 months. This group included a child with Stage IV disease involving the nasal cavity with bony destruction of the left maxilla and metastatic spread to para-aortic nodes and chest wall. He responded well to intensive chemotherapy and radiation therapy and has no evidence of active disease since his initial treatment 12 months ago.

In spite of the limitations of comparison of series of patients from various institutions, the results with this small group of patients indicate that progress is being made in the treatment of non-Hodgkin's lymphoma in children. Radiation therapy in combination with multiple drug chemotherapy and good supportive therapy provides the physician with an increased opportunity to eradicate lymphomas in children, and, in some, to achieve long-term survival without evidence of disease.

REFERENCES

1 WATANABE, A., SULLIVAN, M. P., SUTOW, W. W. and WILBUR, J. R.: Undifferentiated lymphoma, non-Burkitt's type. *Am J Dis Child,* **125:** 57, 1973.

2 BUTLER J. J.: Histopathology of malignant lymphomas and Hodgkin's disease. *In:* Leukemia-Lymphoma: A Collection of Papers Presented at the Fourteenth Annual Clinical Conference on Cancer, 1969, at The University of Texas M. D. Anderson Hospital and Tumor Institute, Houston, Texas. Chicago, Year Book Medical Publishers, Inc. 1970, p.123.

3 ROSENBERG, S. A. *et al.:* Lymphosarcoma in childhood. *N Engl J Med,* **259:** 505, 1958.

4 JENKIN, R. D. T. and SONLEY, M. J.: The management of malignant lymphoma in childhood. *In:* Neoplasia in Childhood: A Collection of Papers Presented at the Twelfth Annual Clinical Conference on Cancer, 1967, at The University of Texas M. D. Anderson Hospital and Tumor Institute, Houston, Texas. Chicago, Year Book Medical Publishers Inc., 1969, p.305.

5 BAILEY, R. J., BURGERT, E. O. and DAHLIN, D. C.: Malignant lymphoma in children. *Pediatrics,* **28:** 985, 1961.

6 JONES, B. *et al.:* Chemotherapy of the leukemic transformation of lymphosarcoma. *J. Pediatr,* **70:** 442, 1967.

7 PIERCE, M. I.: Lymphosarcoma and Hodgkin's disease in children. *In:* Proceedings of the Fourth National Cancer Conference. Philadelphia and Montreal, J. B. Lippincott, 1960, p.559.

BURKITT'S LYMPHOMA

D. P. BURKITT, M.D., M.B., B.Ch., B.A.O., F.R.C.S.(Ed.), Hon. D.Sc.(E.Afr.)*

Before the indentification of the tumor syndrome which subsequently became known as Burkitt's lymphoma, workers in different parts of tropical Africa had recognized an undue prevalence of a number of apparently unconnected tumors in children. These included retinoblastoma, neuroblastoma, sarcomas of the upper and lower jaws and granulosa-cell tumors of the ovary, all of which were composed of small round cells with similar histological appearances. A flaccid paraplegia of rapid onset without evidence of vertebral collapse and tumors of the long bones of the limbs were seen more frequently than might be expected.

It was the simultaneous occurrence of sarcomas in more than one jaw quadrant that first attracted attention, because no pathological process, then known, could have accounted for this bizarre phenomenon.

When attention was focused on these, frequently multiple, jaw tumors, it became evident that they were often associated with other tumors, which had a characteristic anatomical distribution, and appeared to have a predilection for the kidneys, adrenals, ovaries, liver, orbit, salivary glands, testes and thyroid gland. It also became evident that tumors in two or more of these sites tended to occur together in the same individuals even in the absence of jaw involvement. Autopsy evidence revealed that these tumors not only involved multiple anatomical sites but also tended to multifocal involvement of individual organs or structures. Flaccid paralysis of the lower limbs, which could be distinguished from tuberculous paraplegia by the absence of vertebral collapse, was observed to accompany any of these tumors, and the orbital tumors came to be recognized as an upward extension of maxillary neoplasms. These observations indicated that the jaw lesions were not, as at one time considered, primary tumors metastasizing to the other sites.

This close clinical association between tumors in different but characteristic sites suggested that these tumors shared common etiological factors, or that all the tumors were different manifestations of a single disease process – the clinical presentation of which depended on which organ or structure was maximally involved when the patient was first seen. The clinical impression that these tumors were parts of a single disease process was strengthened by finding that the age distribution and geographical distribution of both jaw lesions and

---

***Medical Research Council, London, England.**

other tumors were closely comparable. Meanwhile Davies and O'Conor* had established that these different tumors were indistinguishable histologically and also that the tumor was a lymphoma derived from primitive lymphoid cells. Subsequently, Wright demonstrated that this particular tumor was distinct, histologically and cytologically, from other forms of malignant lymphoma.

The eponym "Burkitt's tumor" was adopted at an International Union Against Cancer (UICC) conference in Paris in 1963, at which time opinion was divided concerning the precise nature of the tumor. There was some disagreement as to whether it was even a "sarcoma", let alone a "lymphoma".

Subsequent studies have established beyond reasonable doubt that the tumor is not only a lymphoma but a specific form of lymphoma, and the more descriptive term "Burkitt's lymphoma" (BL) is now in general use.

FORMULATION OF A HYPOTHESIS

Shortly after this syndrome was recognized it became evident that the tumor was limited to certain geographical areas in Africa. It thus seemed imperative to delineate its geographical distribution and, initially, this task was attempted by postal distribution of an illustrated leaflet and, subsequently, by many extended safaris by land and air in different parts of the continent.

The information thus gleaned indicated that, in Africa, tumor distribution was determined by an altitude barrier above which the disease was rarely, if ever, encountered, and that the critical height fell progressively as the distance from the equator increased. It thus became evident that the altitude barrier reflected a temperature dependence, and that the tumor was only endemic in regions where the temperature did not fall below about 60°F. Similar studies in West Africa, where variations in altitude are small but changes in humidity great, revealed a direct relationship between annual rainfall, with its attendant vegetation pattern, and tumor prevalence. A dry climate was associated with a reduced tumor incidence and *vice versa.*

These observations concerning climatic dependence, which were paralleled by observations in Papua and New Guinea, led Haddow and others to incriminate some biological agent in tumor transmission. Since the geographical distribution of the tumor resembled closely that of many insect-borne diseases, it was postulated that the tumor might be caused by some carcinogenic agent vectored by a species of tropical insect.

---

*A nearly complete list of reference to all aspects of this tumor up till 1970 can be found in "Burkitt's Lymphoma" (1970). Editors, D. P. Burkitt and D. H. Wright, Livingstone, Edinburgh and London.

SEARCH FOR A VIRUS

The only insect-vectored agents known to be carcinogenic, albeit only in animals, were viruses. Therefore, the tumor might be caused by some locally vectored virus, and this supposition stimulated workers in many countries to search for viruses in tumor tissue removed for histological confirmation of a clinical diagnosis.

Various workers made valuable contributions, although some of the viruses isolated were subsequently shown to be unlikely candidates as causative agents. The EB virus first isolated by Epstein and Barr in 1964 from a tissue culture of BL cells has had an exciting subsequent career which merits a book of its own. Sufficient to say that this virus at present appears to be the agent most likely responsible for BL. Not only do all patients with this tumor show high antibody titres to this virus, but immunological cross reactions can be demonstrated between tumor cells from one patient and serum from others.

Following a serendipitous observation by the Henles in Philadelphia, the EB virus was also shown to be the cause of infectious mononucleosis.

MODIFICATION OF A HYPOTHESIS

An examination of the EB virus and further consideration of the world-wide distribution of the tumor impelled a revision of the initial, vectored-virus hypothesis.

Isolated cases of the tumor began to be reported with increasing frequency from all over the world; some regions abounding with presumably suitable insect vectors were apparently tumor-free; the EB virus was not known to be insect vectored; and populations in tumor-endemic regions in Africa showed no higher incidence of EB virus antibodies in their blood than did people in tumor-free areas.

The epidemiology of the tumor was re-evaluated in the light of earlier observations by Dalldorf and O'Conor that hyperendemic or holoendemic malaria might play a causative role. Further studies made it increasingly evident that, in all situations investigated to that time, tumor distribution coincided with that of hyperendemic or holoendemic malaria. Moreover, the only relatively tumor-free areas in tropical Africa were those in which malaria eradication campaigns had been successfully concluded.

The causative relationship between the tumor and intense and persistent malarial infection has been substantiated by a relative immunity afforded against BL by the sickle-cell trait which gives partial protection against falciparum malaria, and by the similarity in geographical distribution between this tumor and some diseases known to be the result of hyperendemic malaria, such as the nephrotic syndrome of children and "big-spleen disease". Moreover animal experiments have shown that mice previously infected with malaria show an increased tendency to develop solid lymphomas with some characteristics similar to human BL.

The hypothesis most consistent with present epidemiological and other evidence is that intense malarial infection depresses the immunological state of the lymphoreticular system and renders its cells more prone to malignant transformation in the presence of the EB or possibly other viruses. Apparently the malarial infection determines the geographical pattern of a disease caused primarily by a ubiquitous virus.

RESPONSE TO THERAPY

An additional and important characteristic of this tumor is its remarkable and sustained response to therapy. With the single exception of choriocarcinoma, which is not a true host tumor, Burkitt's lymphoma is the only form of human cancer in which we can achieve a cure with chemotherapy in a considerable proportion of patients. Moreover, these results can be achieved with relatively non-toxic doses of cytotoxic drugs.

In patients with tumors limited to the jaws, Zeigler, of the National Cancer Institute, and his team working in Uganda recorded approximately 80% long-term survivals, which can be considered probable cures. He had a cure rate of over 50% for all patients excluding those with central nervous system involvement.

The prospect of survival following adequate treatment for tumors detected at an early clinical stage can thus by considered good.

These results are in striking contrast to those achieved with lymphoblastic leukemia in which the tumor cell is closely similar to that of BL. In this instance, dramatic initial response to therapy is followed by almost invariable relapse, and the surviving tumor cells, even if minimal in number, proliferate again to repopulate the temporarily restored marrow. In BL it appears that, following sub-total destruction of unusually sensitive tumor cells by cytotoxic drugs, host-defence mechanisms are competent to deal with the residue.

IMMUNOLOGICAL IMPLICATIONS

As mentioned above, the high rate of long-term remissions, which can be achieved by relatively non-toxic doses of a wide variety of cytotoxic drugs, indicates strong host-defence mechanisms, presumably immunological.

Further evidence for this assumption is provided by well-authenticated reports of spontaneous remission following diagnostic biopsy in patients who have refused treatment, and in patients treated with drugs not known to have any cytotoxic action.

The strong evidence of immunological reactions to this particular tumor has encouraged studies to determine their possible role in other tumors, and similar, though less dramatic evidence, has been found in malignant melanoma.

CURRENT REPERCUSSIONS ON "CANCER" RESEARCH

Sir Harold Himsworth, in his foreword to the monograph "Burkitt's Lymphoma", expressed the opinion that "this tumor may well prove to be something of a Rosetta stone". It would appear to have influenced cancer research in at least the following ways:

a. The fruitfulness of simple epidemiological studies have encouraged similar efforts in the search for a cause of other forms of cancer;

b. The unexpected success achieved with chemotherapy has given renewed hope to workers in this field;

c. If one form of human cancer could be shown to be virus induced, it could be assumed that at least some others have a similar cause;

d. The immunological implications suggest the possible danger of diminishing a patient's own defence mechanisms by overenthusiastic treatment;

e. Perhaps the greatest of all the results of the many studies undertaken on this tumor has been the fostering of friendly communication among workers of different nationalities. All the workers in this field share the credit for what has been achieved, because the work of different individuals or groups could have remained relatively sterile without the complementary contribution of others.

An appraisal of the impact of Burkitt's lymphoma on current cancer research by Graham Bennette in "What We Know About Cancer" may be near the mark.

> "It will probably never be justified to talk about a 'breakthrough' in cancer in the way suggested by some over-enthusiastic reporters, but if ever there were an international communications breakthrough, I think it is Burkitt's tumor that must be seen as the spearhead. From East Africa to London, to Stockholm and Paris, to New York and New Guinea, to Bristol and Philadelphia, to Australia and Minneapolis, and back again to Africa, the dialogues are carried on between every kind of specialist – physicians, radiotherapists, surgeons, pathologists, chemotherapists, virus experts, immunologists, epidemiologists and statisticians. This is an extraordinary phenomenon of communication . . . ."

PANEL ON MALIGNANT LYMPHOMA

Moderator: P. D. McCLURE*
Panelists: C. A. STEPHENS**, J. R. WILBUR†, and D. P. BURKITT‡

Question: Can Dr. Stephens give the age range of the children with Hodgkin's disease subjected to laparotomy and has he seen an increased incidence of septicemia after splenectomy?

Dr. Stephens: One of the 25 children was under the age of 3. Most were in the range 10-17 years. We have not yet seen septicemia in this group of children.

Dr. D'Angio: Recently the American Academy of Pediatric Surgeons circularized a number of surgeons concerning the results of laparotomy in Hodgkin's disease in childhood. In 324 laparotomies they reported 15 children with subsequent intestinal obstruction, of whom 11 required reoperation.

Among 100 of these children who underwent splenectomy, only 13 were less than six years of age, and one of these 13 subsequently died of overwhelming infection. In this experience, one other child, aged 3, also died of sepsis.

Question: One purpose of a laparotomy in Hodgkin's disease is to determine whether the liver is involved. It seems that this is a difficult decision both macroscopically and histologically. Would Dr. Stephens comment?

Dr. Stephens: The liver biopsy was positive histologically in three of the 25 children we subjected to laparotomy. In only one of these did it seem to be involved grossly at the time of operation. In addition, there was a small number in which the pathologist noticed some lymphocytic infiltration in the liver, but which were not classified as being involved with Hodgkin's disease. The three positive patients all had, in addition, a positive spleen and positive retroperitoneal lymph nodes.

Dr. Saunders: In the patients with positive nodes but a negative lymphangiogram, were the positive nodes from areas not shown on the lymphangiogram?

---

*The Hospital for Sick Children, Toronto.
**The Hospital for Sick Children, Toronto.
†Children's Cancer Unit. Children's Hospital at Stanford, Palo Alto, California, U.S.A.
‡Medical Research Council, London, England.

Dr. Stephens: I do not have that correlation. Certainly some of the positive nodes were from the celiac region or splenic hilus – areas that would not have been demonstrable by lymphangiography.

Question: Can Dr. Burkitt tell us how long he was in Africa before appreciating the unusual nature of his tumor?

Dr. Burkitt: I was in Africa 11 years, totally blind to this tumor. Sometimes I feel like the little boy who planned to boil an egg but instead set fire to the prairie.

Dr. Schweisguth: Would Dr. Wilbur tell us a little more about his experience with exploratory laparotomy in non-Hodgkin's lymphoma in childhood?

Dr. Wilbur: We have carried out this procedure in only five or six children. Two had disease, which had not been recognized during their previous investigation. The children all had Stage I or II disease clinically. It seems to me that in a small group of children with non-Hodgkin's lymphoma and apparently regional disease, positive findings at laparotomy could influence treatment by indicating the best way of combining irradiation and chemotherapy.

Question: North American Burkitt's lymphoma does not seem to respond clinically like this disease in Africa. Is this the same tumor?

Dr. Burkitt: Criteria, other than histological, are needed to make this diagnosis. In particular, the EB virus antibody titre may be of help. In Africa, results are better in those areas where this lymphoma is common than where it is uncommon. In the areas where it is common, it occurs more often at an earlier age and more often affects the facial bones, so that many factors seem to be involved in prognosis.

Dr. Dent: I would like to emphasize that the immunological status is changed after splenectomy and that this change will be important beyond the first two to three years of life. Thus, these patients do have some partial impairment of their immunological competence. In particular, phagocytosis may be altered, and the splenic component of IgM antibody production is lost.

CONTROLLED CLINICAL TRIALS IN LEUKEMIA IN CHILDREN

L. F. SINKS, M.D.*

Clinicians have long been plagued by the difficulty of distinguishing between effective and noneffective therapy in rare diseases. In the not too distant past, most reports of effectiveness under these conditions can best be described as anecdotal. To overcome some of these defects, Holland, Frei, Zubrod and other interested physicians combined in 1956 to form the Acute Leukemia Group B. The major objectives of this co-operative chemotherapy group were:

1. To enable physicians to treat and study a greater number of patients with rare diseases in a shorter period through a predetermined method;
2. To enable rapid exploitation of animal model systems in man;
3. To shorten the time needed to test well-established drugs with respect to both dose and interval;
4. To facilitate the rapid exploration of the newer chemotherapeutic agents in the treatment of malignant disease.

While all recognized that the true etiology of acute leukemia of childhood was still unknown, there was sufficient reason to believe that available therapy could cure this disease. However, such cure required the co-operative approach.

In 1963, Selawry[1] wrote Protocol No. 6307 and brought to clinical application an animal model system tested by Golden *et al.* The latter observed that mice with L1210 leukemia responded better to methotrexate (MTX) given every fourth day, rather than to daily administration. It has been conventional for clinicians to treat leukemic children with MTX on a daily basis ever since Farber and colleagues introduced the antifolic agents in 1948[2]. Previous studies had shown that the combination of vincristine (VCR) and prednisone (Pred) induced remissions in 85% of children with acute lymphoblastic leukemia, but were not suitable for use as maintenance agents[3]. Selawry's study was designed to treat all children initially with the combination of VCR and Pred. As soon as a remission was achieved, one-half of the children would be randomized to a maintenance regimen consisting of 30 mg./m^2 of MTX given intramuscularly every four days, and the other one-half would receive MTX 3 mg./m^2 daily by mouth. This simple study was rewarded because it showed the vast superiority of twice-weekly MTX over daily administration. The median remission on the twice-weekly regimen was about 17 months and the median remission on the

*Roswell Park Memorial Institute, Buffalo, New York, U.S.A.

daily dose was 3.3 months. Subsequently, others demonstrated that the route of administration had little to do with the superior results and that one could administer MTX in high doses twice weekly by mouth and achieve results comparable to the intramuscular route. This study is a clear example of the effectiveness of a co-operative study in exploiting animal model systems at the clinical level. It also demonstrates the importance of dose levels and intervals of administration.

In 1966, a direct sequel of 6307 involved repeated five-day courses of intravenous MTX at varying dose schedules of 12, 15 and 18 mg./m^2. Children brought into successful remission with VCR and Pred would receive three five-day courses of intravenous MTX at one of the dose levels. Subsequently, they were randomized to one of four maintenance schedules. One group was to be on no maintenance (control – Schedule A), a second group received twice-weekly MTX (Schedule B), a third group (Schedule C) was to continue with five-day courses of intravenous MTX. The fourth group of children would receive periodic inducer doses of VCR and Pred (Schedule D).

The survival of these children was clearly dose dependent. Those receiving 18 mg./m^2 intravenously survived longest. It is apparent that the length of remission was affected by the type of maintenance therapy. Children receiving the Schedule D had longer remissions than those in the other regimens. The influence of the inducer doses of VCR and Pred was clearly evident.

After the completion of Study 6601, a subsequent study (No. 6801) in 1968, was stimulated by the observations of Professor Bernard and colleagues at the *Institute de Recherches sur les Leucemies* in Paris. Recently, this study was terminated when it included 514 children. Originally, No. 6801 was intended to compare the inductive capacity of VCR and daunorubicin (DNR) *plus* Pred with the conventional VCR and Pred combination. However, approximately a year after the study was begun, accumulated experience with L-asparaginase (L-ASP)[4] suggested that we should incorporate L-ASP as a preinductive course before conventional therapy. Upon completion of induction, various maintenance regimens were then to be tested (Fig. 1).

Equally important was the decision to test the hypothesis: does prophylactic intrathecal MTX prevent the development of central-nervous-system leukemia? To answer this question, one-half of the children were given intrathecal MTX 12 mg./m^2 at the same time they received the pulse dose of VCR, DNR and Pred. The other one-half of the children were followed without central-nervous-system therapy.

To date, the results of this study are extremely provocative. The addition of DNR to the induction regimen does not increase the proportion of children induced or prolong the duration of remission (Fig. 2). Moreover, the use of L-ASP before conventional induction therapy does not appear to increase the proportion of children going into remission, or increase the duration of remission.

STUDY DESIGN FOR PROTOCOL ALGB #6801

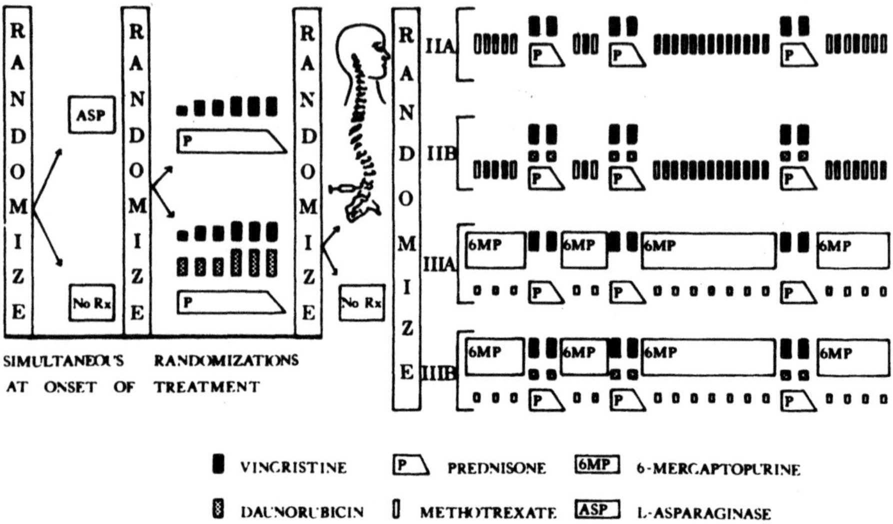

Fig. 1. *First Randomization:* Black indicates L-asparaginase (L-ASP) 1000 units/kg. x 5 days, blank indicates *no* L-ASP.

Second Randomization: Solid bar indicates prednisone (Pred.) 120 mg./m^2 by mouth daily during induction, vertical bar indicates vincristine 2 mg./m^2 I.V. once each week; 2nd row of bars indicates daunorubicin (DNR) 60 mg./m^2.

Third Randomization: This indicates that 50% of the patients were allocated to receive preventive intrathecal (IT) methotrexate (MTX) 12 mg./m^2 with each dose of VCR during induction and with each pulse dose during maintenance. The other 50% were to have only a lumbar puncture.

Fourth Randomization: IIa light vertical bars indicate biweekly MTX 30 mg./m^2 p.o. Heavy vertical bars indicate VCR pulse dose 2 mg./m^2. Heavy horizontal bar indicates Pred. 120 mg./m^2 for 7 days. IIb identical to IIa, but the small heavy blocks indicate DNR 60 mg./m^2 added to pulse doses. IIIa light bar indicates 6-mercaptopurine (6-MP) 90 mg./m^2 p.o. qd. Light vertical bar indicates MTX 15 mg./m^2 p.o. once weekly. Pulse doses. as indicated in IIa, IIIb, are identical to IIIa but the small heavy blocks indicate DNR 60 mg./m^2 is added to pulse doses.

Schedule of Pulse Doses: VCR given once monthly for six months during maintenance along with seven days of Pred. DNR is given simultaneously when added to pulse doses of VCR and Pred. At six months. two doses of VCR or VCR/DNR are given at seven-day intervals; at nine months. two doses are again given; at 12 months, three doses of VCR or VCR/DNR are given at seven-day intervals; then VCR or VCR/DNR are repeated every six months.

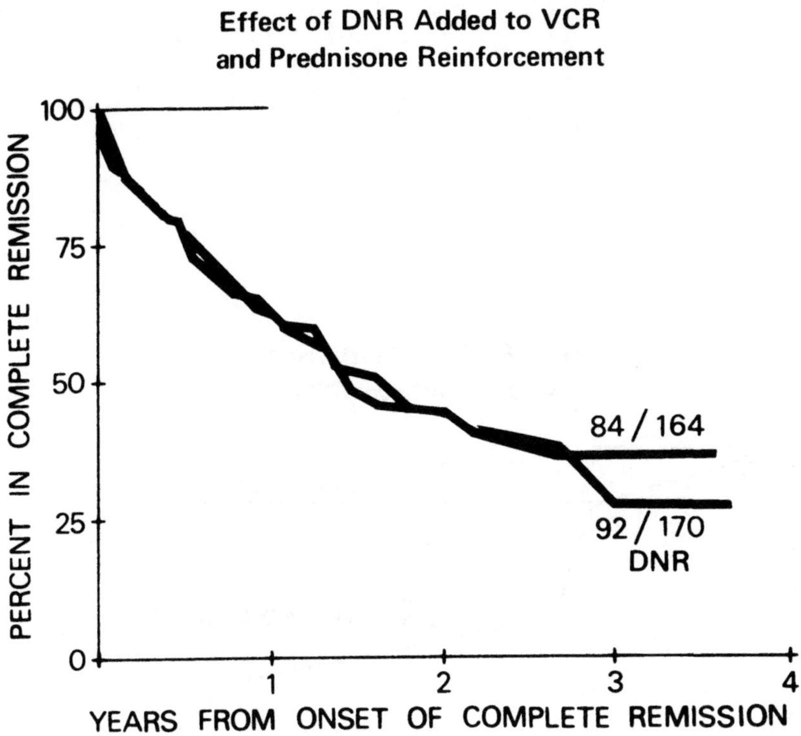

Fig. 2. The curve identified as DNR indicates patients received pulse doses (reinforcement) of VCR, DNR and Pred. The control curve indicates the remission curve of patients receiving only VCR and Pred pulse doses.

The longer duration of remission of children induced with VCR and Pred and treated with intrathecal MTX followed by the maintenance schedule of 6-mercaptopurine (6-MP) daily, once weekly MTX and monthly inducer doses of VCR and Pred is clearly evident in Fig. 3.

However, it should be emphasized that 10% of children who received maintenance DNR developed severe cardiac toxicity, which killed several of them while they were in complete remission[5].

Study 6801 has demonstrated:

1. DNR does not increase the proportion of children induced into remission; nor does it prolong the remission time when used as a reinforcement dose;
2. L-asparaginase given during the induction period (as described) does not increase the proportion of patients induced nor prolong remission;
3. Intrathecal methotrexate does protect the patient from developing CNS leukemia;
4. Ninety per cent of children induced with VCR and Pred, given IT MTX and maintained with 6-MP and once weekly MTX, plus doses (reinforcement) of VCR and Pred are living for 36 months.

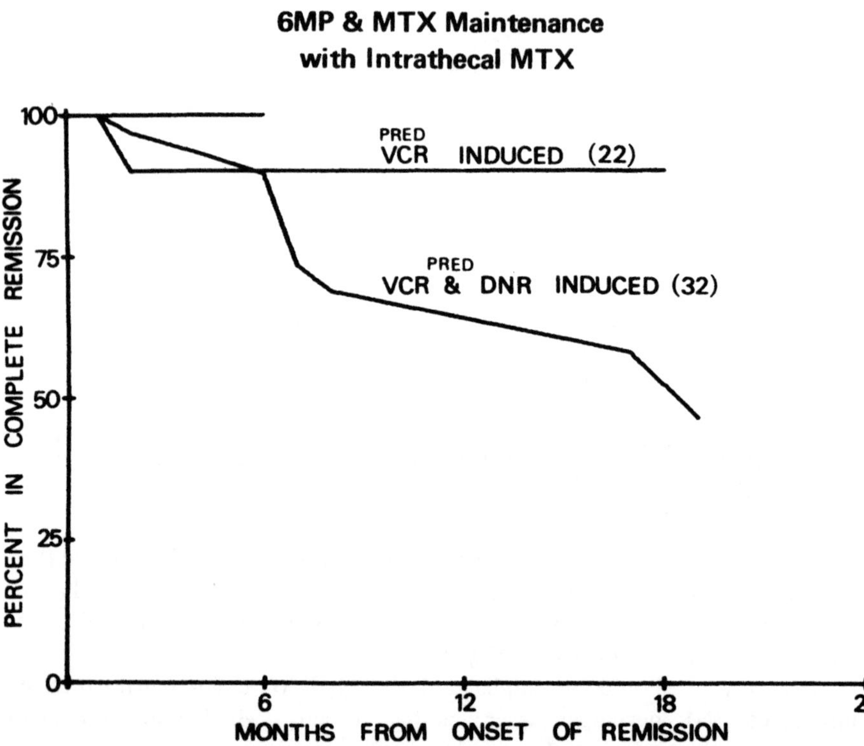

Fig. 3. Remission duration of patients receiving maintenance of 6-MP and MTX, as well as preventive IT MTX. The influence of the two types of induction therapy is noted.

In summary, Figs. 4, 5, and 6 show how the average survival and duration of remission has increased over the last decade. It is also interesting to note that the proportion of five-year survivors has increased substantially during this same period.

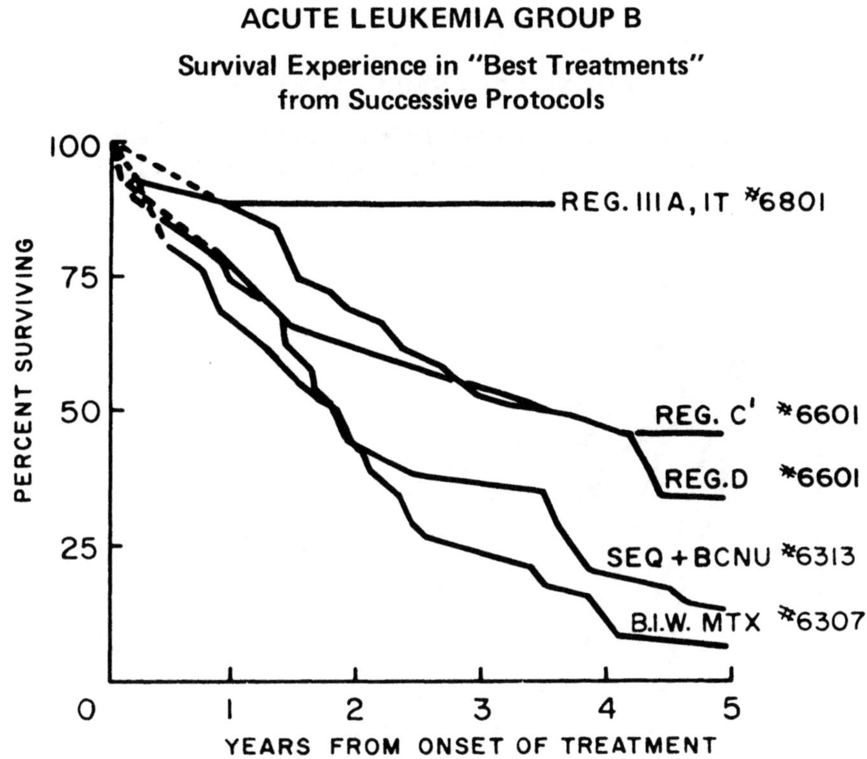

Fig. 4. Survival of children in relationship to best treatment schedule from studies commencing in 1963 until 1968 (first two figures in designation refers to year of study.)

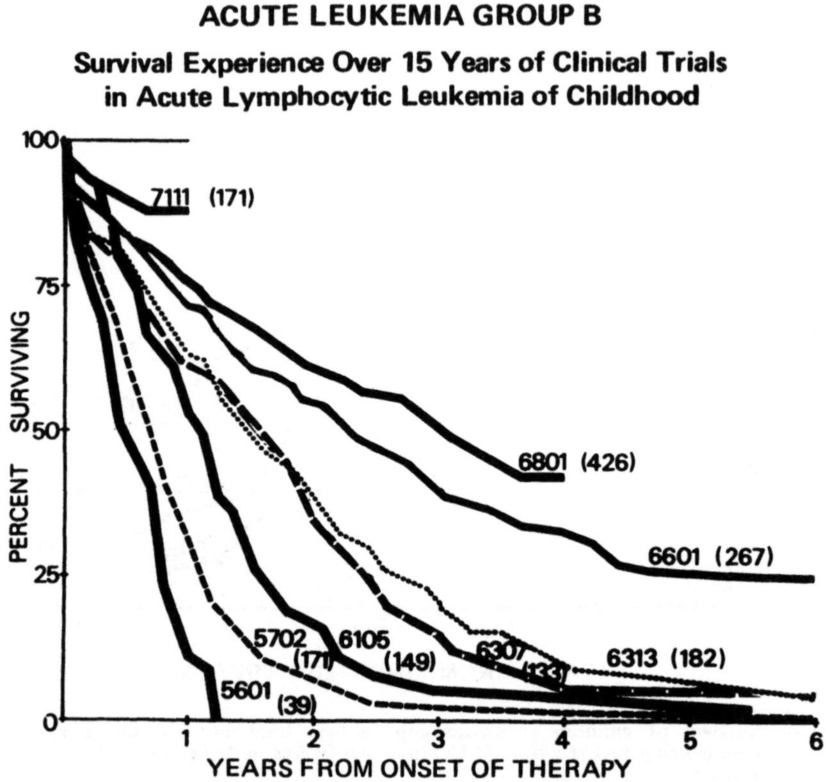

Fig. 5. Overall survival of children with acute leukemia in relationship to studies commencing in 1956 through 1971.

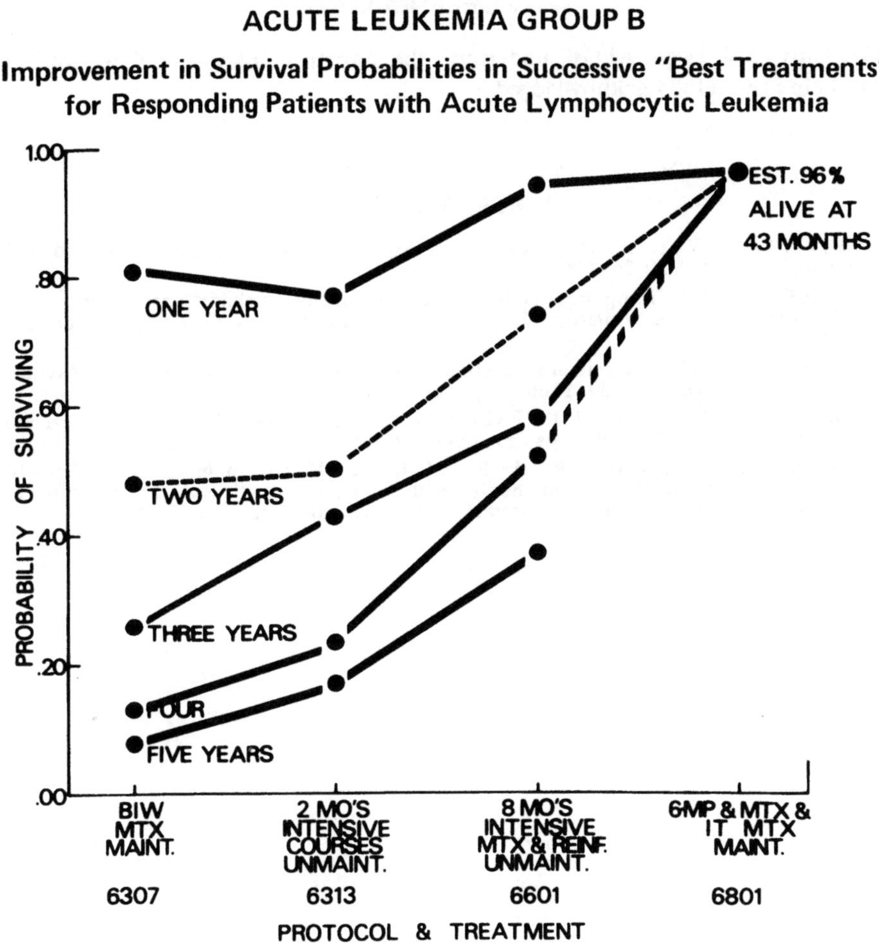

Fig. 6. The survival expressed as proportion of patients living for one, two, three, four and five years in relationship to best treatment schedule of the various studies commencing in 1963.

We anticipate that approximately 35% of the children on No. 6801 will survive five years and that present studies will still further improve the treatment of this disease.

ACKNOWLEDGEMENT

Dr. Oliver Glidewell, ALGB, undertook the statistical analysis of these studies. His help is gratefully acknowledged.

REFERENCES

1 SELAWRY, O. S., *et al.*: New treatment schedule with improved survival in childhood leukemia. *JAMA*, **194**: 75, 1965.

2 FARBER, S., *et al.*: Temporary remission in acute leukemia in children produced by folic acid antagonist, 4-aminopteroyl glutamic acid (aminopterin). *N Engl J Med*, **238**: 787, 1948.

3 KARON, M., *et al.*: The role of vincristine in the treatment of childhood acute leukemia. *Clin Pharmacol Ther*, **7**: 332, 1966.

4 OHNUMA, T., HOLLAND, J. R., FREEMAN, A. I. and SINKS, L. F.: Biochemical and pharmacological studies with asparaginase in man. *Cancer Res*, **30**: 2297, 1970.

5 HALAZUN, J. F., WAGNER, H. R., SINKS, L. F. and Members of ALGB: II. Daunorubicin cardiac toxicity in children with acute lymphocytic leukemia. Presented at the XIV International Congress of Hematology, Sao Paulo, Brazil, July 16-22, 1972.

VIRAL INFECTIONS IN ACUTE LEUKEMIA

PETER J. MIDDLETON, M.D., F.R.C.P.A.*

In both our local experience and in the literature, the herpes group of viruses (especially varicella zoster) are the main virus pathogens in patients receiving immunosuppressive therapy and/or who have lymphoma or leukemia. Other viruses, which produce florid disease in this class of patients, include the pox group, i.e., vaccinia and molluscum contagiosum; the papovoviruses represented by warts, and the agent(s) associated with the progressive multifocal leukoencephalopathy; and measles virus in the paramyxo group. Rubella, arbovirus, rhino and enterovirus infections appear to be tolerated reasonably well.

DIAGNOSIS

In the group of patients under discussion the establishment of a specific virological diagnosis should prove no more difficult than in the conventional patient, if simple guidelines are observed in taking adequate specimens at appropriate times during the virus illness. Moreover, certain of these specimens must be properly preserved for delivery to a virus laboratory, e.g., urine for cytomegalovirus isolation must be brought to pH7.0 after collection and delivered promptly without freezing or chilling.

When the patient suffers from an obvious, clearly identifiable virus disease, the taking of the most appropriate specimen and the ability to make a positive virus diagnosis should present no great problem. When, however, the patient exhibits a less clear-cut syndrome or the illness has been present for a week or longer, virological investigations are usually much less precise and rewarding. In this situation, diagnosis depends on factors which determine not only the specimen(s) collected but also the procedures to be performed in the laboratory. These factors are: the clinical syndrome, season of the year, age of the patient, preceding events, e.g., vaccination or prodromal illness, geographical locality, whether the syndrome is epidemic or sporadic in the community, epidemiological information from adjacent centres doing virological work, and exclusion of other non-viral conditions. Only after he has considered these various factors, is it possible for the physician to arrive at a differential virus diagnosis. Armed with a list of possible virus pathogens, appropriate specimens are collected and laboratory procedures initiated to identify the suspected virus.

---

*Chief of Virology, The Hospital for Sick Children, Toronto; Associate Professor of Medical Microbiology, University of Toronto; and Assistant Professor of Microbiology, School of Hygiene, University of Toronto.

The virus laboratory usually mounts a three-pronged attack on such problems: virus isolation, antibody studies, and demonstration of virus or virus antigen. Serological studies alone are often not conclusive because of previous virus infections, heterologous responses to the antigen, and low-grade or even negative responses to antigenic stimulation. Moreover, an answer is often delayed because two serum samples must be collected at intervals of at least one week. These factors combine to make antibody studies the most undesirable approach. Virus isolation, while more precise, also has certain drawbacks. Both cytomegalovirus and varicella-zoster viruses usually take more than seven days to produce a recognizable cytopathic effect. In some instances, isolation of a virus from nasopharyngeal secretions or feces does not necessarily implicate that specific virus as the agent responsible for the disease in that patient. Now with accurate immunofluorescence microscopy and the electron microscope, the physician can often have a definitive diagnosis on the same day the specimen is submitted. "Same-day" diagnosis confers the obvious advantage of providing prompt and appropriate patient management. In addition, it permits the physician to institute prophylactic measures in contacts who may also be at high risk. Herpes simplex and varicella-zoster infections can be readily distinguished from one another either by immunofluorescence or by first examining the specimen under electron microscopy to establish that the virus is a member of the herpes group; if it is, cell cultures are then inoculated with the specimen(s). By the next day, a herpes simplex virus should produce a cytopathic effect whereas varicella-zoster or cytomegalovirus will not. While we have had no success in making a diagnosis of measles from examining nasopharyngeal secretions under direct electron microscopy, we have shown that, by modifying the usual indirect immunofluorescence test, we can make a positive diagnosis up to four days after the onset of rash. Once the rash of measles has been present for longer than 24 hours, it is usually not possible to isolate measles virus as local antibody produced by the patient has inactivated any free virus.

PREVENTION – PROPHYLAXIS – TREATMENT

Segregation and isolation in the hospital and in the home may help to slow or stop the spread of infection to patients who are at particular risk because they are receiving immunosuppressive therapy or have lymphoma or leukemia, but these measures frequently break down because the virus has usually disseminated before the contacts exhibit signs or symptoms of disease. The new policy concerning small pox vaccination probably will reduce the number of patients who develop complications after contact with vaccinia virus. Development of "herd" immunity by widespread community vaccination, as now practised for mumps, rubella and measles may reduce circulating virus in the community, and thereby lessen the chance of spread to patients with leukemia.

Prophylaxis can be attained either by a prospective approach or through problem-based efforts, e.g., an immunosuppressed child with a very recent history of chicken pox contact is given either zoster immune globulin or cytosine arabinoside. At the Hospital for Sick Children, Toronto, although we have not adopted prospective prophylaxis in our patients with leukemia, we have for some time regularly surveyed (at three to six monthly intervals) those who are on, or who may come onto the renal dialysis program. Our regular periodic serological studies provide exclusion diagnoses at a time when the patient becomes ill, e.g., previous measles infection; in addition, these studies give us the option of administering appropriate vaccinations when the patient has no immunity to a particular virus. These surveys also identify those patients who are likely to become infected or reinfected with a particular virus. However, it would be a formidable undertaking to maintain serological surveillance of the much greater number of patients with leukemia, Hodgkin's disease, and/or who are on immunosuppressive regimens.

Passive immunization using human immune serum globulin up to a week post-exposure has proved its value in preventing measles infection, but has not given encouraging results in mumps and rubella. Zoster-immune globulin (ZIG) appears to be valuable in preventing or modifying varicella, even in subjects with compromised immune mechanisms. The pyrimidine nucleoside, cytosine arabinoside, which acts by inhibiting a step in virus-DNA elaboration, may also be used for varicella prophylaxis.

The management and specific treatment of patients with severe virus disease who in addition may also have varying degrees of immunodepression is confused by the fact that we know very little concerning the various specific parameters of the host defence system, e.g., we do not know why recurrent herpes simplex infections are resolved. In the meantime, until we learn more about the relative importance of interferon, cellular immunity and antibody response in the resolution of different virus infections in patients with different diseases, we will have to rely on a few rather toxic virostatic drugs now available. These include N-methylisatin β-thiosemicarbazone for pox virus infections, plus pyrimidine and purine nucleosides, e.g., 5-iodo-2-deoxyuridine, cytosine arabinoside, adenine arabinoside, which are used mainly for the herpes viruses. The exact role and usefulness of rifampin, polyinosinic-polycytidylic acid and virazole (a synthetic nucleoside) have yet to be determined.

SUMMARY

Significant virus disease among immunodepressed and immunosupressed patients usually involves herpes simplex, varicella-zoster, cytomegalovirus, vaccinia, measles, the agent(s) associated with progressive multifocal leukoencephalopathy plus certain respiratory viruses.

When appropriate laboratory investigations employing sensitive detection systems are pursued early in the course of illness, offending virus may often be demonstrated.

Vaccination programs for those at risk and of the "herd" together with isolation and segregation measures, provide the basis of current preventive measures. For the prophylaxis of contacts either high-titred specific globulin or an antiviral drug may be used. The actual treatment of established virus disease is handicapped by a limited range of somewhat toxic drugs and our lack of understanding of the relative importance of the various parameters underlying the host defense system in different types of virus infection.

BACTERIAL INFECTION IN LEUKEMIA

P. C. FLEMING, M.B., B.S., M.R.C.S., L.R.C.P., M.R.C.Path. (Eng.)*

Levine, Graw and Young[1] recently reviewed all aspects of the problem of infection in leukemia, and Hughes[2], in a series of 200 fatal cases of childhood leukemia, found that death was due to infection in 45% and that it was a contributing factor in another 35%. Thus, in the latter series, infection was a significant factor in the demise in 80% of children with leukemia. A common feature of infection is the rise in temperature, and it has been estimated that, in acute leukemias, between 60 and 80% of all febrile reactions are due to this cause. Infection is much more common in the presence of neutropenia and, when below 500 neutrophils per cu. mm. and particularly when this has persisted over one month, approximately 90% of these children will develop infection. In this situation, children do not develop the usual purulent reaction and may not even have the expected radiographic signs. Therefore, a fever, especially in a neutropenic individual, must be regarded as due to infection until proved otherwise. Blood cultures and all other relevant specimens should be collected and treatment commenced immediately.

For the first two to four days, treatment will need to be blind while awaiting the results of the blood and other cultures and the sensitivities of isolated organisms. Newer techniques for detecting the presence of bacterial growth by demonstrating metabolic products derived from radioactive substrates incorporated in culture media, promise to reduce this time to a few hours[3]. However, at the moment, these techniques are experimental and expensive.

Concerning the causative organisms, most institutes now find that, of the bacteria, *Pseudomonas aeruginosa* is the most common and accounts for about 50% of isolations. This is closely followed by *Escherichia coli* and, with some variation in frequency, by other members of the Enterobacteriaceae family, such as the Klebsiellae and the members of the *Proteus genus. Staphylococcus aureus* and hemolytic streptococcal infections are still seen but are not nearly as common as the gram-negative isolates.

Fungal infections are not common in "fresh" leukemic patients but become more so with longer survival periods, particularly after two years. Over 90% of such infections are likely to be due to *Candida albicans.*

Pneumonia due to a probable protozoan, *Pneumocystis carinii,* is also seen later in the disease and, paradoxically, tends to become manifest while the child is in a state of remission, often following methotrexate therapy.

---

*Bacteriologist-in-Chief, The Hospital for Sick Children, Toronto; Professor, Medical Microbiology, and Assistant Professor of Pediatrics, University of Toronto.

Four antibiotics, carbenicillin, cephalothin, gentamicin and clindamycin may be used together (Table I) until the etiological agent and its "antibiogram" are determined.

TABLE I

Childhood Leukemia:
Antibiotic Combination for Treatment of Febrile Episodes
(Modified after Tattersall et al.[8])

Carbenicillin	–	500-1000 mg./kg./day I.V.	divided every 6 hr.
Cephalothin	–	200 mg./kg./day I.V.	
Gentamicin	–	3-6 mg./kg./day I.V.	divided every 8 hr.
Clindamycin	–	20 mg./kg./day I.V. or by mouth	

Use lower dose of gentamicin if serum levels are not monitored regularly. Administer penicillins and cephalosporins rapidly followed by infusion of gentamicin over a one-hour period.

Carbenicillin and gentamicin, both bactericidal drugs, are used to cover the probability of pseudomonas infection. It is important that both agents are used together because the organism may be resistant or relatively insensitive to either separately. In addition, this combination has been shown to have a synergistic activity against 50% of strains of *Pseudomonas aeruginosa.* This regimen is likely to be much more effective than polymyxin or colistimethanesulphonate for parenteral pseudomonas infections. Indeed, it is doubtful if the latter drugs should now be used in this situation.

While each dose of carbenicillin and cephalothin should be administered rapidly (within 5-30 minutes), it is most important that each dose of gentamicin be infused over a period of close to one hour's duration to avoid dangerous peak levels or continuous but ineffective low levels. The penicillin and cephalosporins inactivate gentamicin *in vitro,* therefore, the latter should not be mixed in the same intravenous fluid with carbenicillin or cephalothin.

The high dose of gentamicin should not be used for more than 48 hours unless the serum levels are being monitored, and peak levels of 12 μg./ml. should not be exceeded. Serum levels can be determined from capillary samples with as little as 35 microlitres of blood, and the results reported within four to six hours even in the presence of other antibiotics. However, many anomalous results have been reported because the physician has failed to report to the laboratory relevant facts concerning recent or concurrent antibiotic chemotherapy. Repeated doses of gentamicin should not be given to patients with impaired renal function unless serum levels are monitored or the clearance of the drug can otherwise be accurately calculated. Too high a level of the drug may induce vestibular dysfunction or, more rarely, permanent hearing loss.

Because of the wide range in the amount of carbenicillin required to kill different strains of pseudomonas, a high dosage must be used (500 to 1000 mg./kg./day). Although the drug is normally considered non-toxic, at this level it may interfere with platelet aggregation and may prolong the bleeding time[4]. This effect is not likely to be important in leukemic episode but an awareness of it may help the physician to interpret unusual hematological findings.

The combination of gentamicin and cephalothin should cover most other infections due to the different members of the Enterobacteriaceae, and, in many instances, the combination again has a synergistic effect.

The combined activity of cephalothin and clindamycin will provide excellent "cover" against staphylococcal and streptococcal infections, and, in addition, the latter is likely to cover members of the Bacteroides group, which are anaerobic and sometimes missed.

This aggressive form of therapy, if quickly instituted, should give the child adequate protection until an organism is isolated and definitive therapy can be chosen. If the child shows no clinical response by 72 hours and the blood cultures are negative, he probably has no bacteriological infection and there would seem to be no need to continue the regimen.

If the child has evidence of superficial candidiasis infection and there is evidence or strong suspicion of parenteral invasion, systemic amphotericin B remains the drug of choice. A persisting progressive pneumonia, in spite of antibacterial chemotherapy, should raise the suspicion of pneumocystis infection, particularly if these signs develop in a child in remission. It is as yet difficult to demonstrate the existence of pneumocystis pneumonia by identifying the organism in bronchoscopic aspirates although this is sometimes possible. More often a lung biopsy is necessary for certain proof. For treatment, the course of pentamidine (4 mg./kg./day) should last for two weeks and no response should be expected for at least five days.

Inasmuch as the main portal of entry of the infecting Enterobacteriaceae may be the ulcers so frequently present in the gastrointestinal tract in acute leukemia, those children particularly at risk have been treated prophylactically by reducing the gut flora by the systematic oral administration of non-absorbable antibiotics. Usually combinations of aminoglycoside antibiotics with a polymyxin or sulphonamide are rotated to delay the emergence of resistant organisms[5]. We have found that children do not tolerate this system well and are not using it at the moment. A better prophylactic regimen may be that outlined in Table II. It seems desirable to reduce the child's exposure to the sometimes heavy loads of pseudomonas and other Enterobacteriaceae, which are often present in various foodstuffs by ensuring that the food is cooked and, hence, heated to the required levels.

TABLE II

Prophylactic Regimen for Gut Sterilization (From Levine et al.[1])

Gentamicin	–	200 mg. four times daily (qid)
Vancomycin	–	500 mg. qid
Nystatin	–	3 million units qid

When used in association with a cooked food program and/or isolation program, this program reduces sepsis.

Gentamicin levels should be monitored by serum measurements.

Colonization resistance in the bowel is probably decreased in patients with acute leukemia and therefore they are apt to be host to many more different strains of Enterobacteriaceae than normal individuals[6]. Nursing in strict isolation should reduce the number of such strains, which are constantly derived from exogenous sources. Thus, if patients can be decontaminated or rendered "specific-pathogen free" by appropriate chemotherapy, it is theoretically possible to maintain them in this state. However, this requires special units, exacting procedures and specially trained nursing and medical staffs. It is questionable whether this complex procedure is worthwhile if the predisposing leukemia cannot be adequately treated. It is, however, comforting to know that if a breakthrough is achieved in leukemia, such isolation systems can work and that their efficiency can now be demonstrated by reliable methods[1,6,7]

REFERENCES

1 LEVINE, A. S., GRAW, R. G. Jr. and YOUNG, R. C.: Management of infections in patients with leukemia and lymphoma: Current concepts and experimental approaches. *Semin Hematol*, 9: 141, 1972.

2 HUGHES, W. T.: Fatal infections in childhood leukaemia. *Am J Dis Child*, 122: 283, 1971.

3 DeBLANC, H. J., DELAND, F. and WAGNER, H. W.: Automated radiometric detection of bacteria in 2967 blood cultures. *Appl Microbiol*, 22: 846, 1971.

4 McCLURE, P. D., CASSERLEY, J., MONSIER, C. and CROZIER, D. N.: Carbenicillin induced bleeding disorder. *Lancet*, II: 1307, 1970.

5 PREISLER, H. D., GOLDSTEIN, I. M. and HENDERSON, E. S.: Gastrointestinal "sterilization" in the treatment of patients with acute leukemia. *Cancer*, 26: 1076, 1970.

6 WAAIJ, D. VAN DER and SPELTIE, T. M.: Biotyping of enterobacteriaceae as a test for the evaluation of isolation systems. *J Hyg (Camb)*, 70: 639, 1972.

7 SOLBERG, C. O., MATSEN, J. M., VESLEY, D., WHEELER, D. J., GOOD, R. A. and MEUWISSEN, H. J.: Laminar airflow protection in bone marrow transplantation. *Appl Microbiol*, 21: 209, 1971.

8 TATTERSALL, M. H., SPIERS, A. S. and DARRELL, J. H.: Initial therapy with combination of five antibiotics in febrile patients with leukaemia and neutropenia. *Lancet*, 1: 162, 1972.

METHOTREXATE TOXICITY

M. H. FREEDMAN, M. D., F.R.C.P.(C)*

After more than 20 years of clinical use, methotrexate has shown itself to be an effective and versatile chemotherapeutic agent. By its antifolate action, it impairs the synthesis of deoxyribonucleic acid (DNA) and ribonucleic acid (RNA), an action that accounts for its clinical usefulness as well as its toxicity.

Generally speaking, methotrexate is a reasonably safe drug, but toxicity is common, and becomes evident in the following circumstances: with overdosage; with prolonged intravenous infusion; with intrathecal installation (which, in effect, is the same as a prolonged intravenous infusion); when used in combination with x-radiation or other antineoplastic drugs; and, finally, for no explainable reason, in patients who, possibly on a pharmacogenetic basis, are exquisitely sensitive to small doses of the drug.

The toxic effects can be divided into two general groups: those that occur commonly, and those that are infrequent and unusual (Table I).

TABLE I

Toxicity of Methotrexate

COMMON:	UNCOMMON:
Gastrointestinal	Pulmonary ("methotrexate lung")
Bone marrow suppression	Hepatic
Immunosuppression	Skeletal
	Neurologic
	Dermatologic

Of the common toxic effects, gastrointestinal manifestations head the list. Aside from nausea and vomiting, mouth ulcers appear early and are often the only sign of toxicity. They usually predate more severe toxicity and provide a cue for the clinician to reduce the dosage or stop the drug. The lips, tongue and palate are the usual sites but the ulcers may extend through the entire gut and produce abdominal pain, bloody stools, ileus, and even perforation. Folinic acid, given in at least one-quarter of any large dose of methotrexate within two to 36 hours, will prevent acute toxicity such as mouth ulcers.

---

*The Hospital for Sick Children, Toronto, Ontario.

The typical megaloblastic changes in red-cell precursors induced by methotrexate, which can often be detected in the bone marrow even though the peripheral blood counts are normal, are considered to be a mild sign of drug effect. More severe toxicity is associated with pancytopenia secondary to marrow suppression.

Another common toxic effect is immunosuppression. This predisposes the child, not only to persistent upper respiratory illness but also to infections seen in those whose host resistance is lowered, namely, bacteremia, *pneumocystis carinii* pneumonia, severe systemic viremia, acquired toxoplasmosis and generalized fungus infections. It is the usual practice to stop the drug while treating such infections.

A number of uncommon toxic effects have been described recently. The first of these is a pulmonary disease syndrome[1] known familiarly as "methotrexate lung". Characteristically it occurs 12 to 100 days after the start of methotrexate in patients with acute leukemia in remission. A dry cough, fever, dyspnea and peripheral eosinophilia have been reported in most cases. The typical chest film shows bilateral diffuse interstitial pulmonary infiltrates, often marked at the bases, with patchy areas of consolidation in severe cases. Open lung biopsy on one patient showed an intra-alveolar and interstitial granulomatous lesion composed of epithelioid cells, giant cells, lymphocytes and eosinophils. All appropriate microbiological cultures in these patients are negative. The acute phase of the illness usually lasts 10 to 40 days and then clears, regardless of whether methotrexate therapy is continued or not.

Methotrexate-induced liver disease[2] has been suspected since 1955 when a high incidence of cirrhosis was noted in autopsies of children with acute leukemia who had received large doses of methotrexate. Also an increasing number of cases have been reported in patients receiving methotrexate for psoriasis. A liver biopsy from such a patient showed multiple nodules of hepatic parenchyma divided by thin, fibrous septae, and inflammatory infiltrate in the portal areas. A high-power view showed pleomorphism of hepatic cells with large, irregular nuclei and vacuolar fat. Liver destruction may proceed even after stopping the drug because it is stored in hepatic tissue for weeks to months. Standard liver function tests often do not reflect the severity of such liver damage.

Bony changes have been reported in children with acute leukemia, in remission, while on long-term methotrexate therapy[3]. Clinically, there may be mild to severe bone pain which can mimic leukemia in relapse. This, as well as the radiographic changes, improve after stopping the drug. The radiographic features include growth disturbance lines, mild to severe osteoporosis and fractures. The knees of a five-year-old boy with acute leukemia in remission, for example, showed osteoporosis which closely resembled scurvy. Bony repair was demonstrated four months after chemotherapy was stopped.

The drug has neurologic toxic effects[4]. Seven patients have been described in whom an encephalopathy developed after prolonged courses of methotrexate, in part by intrathecal injection. The main features are confusion, irritability, somnolence, tremor, ataxia and fits. In one death reported in the literature the autopsy showed numerous small infarcts in brain tissue without evidence of active leukemic disease or of viral encephalitis. The condition did not respond to radiotherapy. On the other hand, improvement was reported after the drug was stopped and the patient was given folinic acid.

Lastly, some dermatologic effects may occur. Perifolliculitis, vesiculation, photosensitivity reaction, generalized itchy macular rash, and alopecia have all been reported after methotrexate therapy.

In summary, the drug commonly has gastrointestinal effects, notably mouth ulcers, peripheral blood changes, and an increased tendency to infection due to the immunosuppressive action.

Less commonly, but especially when the drug is used on a long-term basis, the attending physician should be alert to the pulmonary, hepatic, skeletal and neurologic syndromes that are occasionally seen.

REFERENCES

1 CLARYSSE, A. M., *et al.:* Pulmonary disease complicating intermittent therapy with methotrexate. *JAMA,* **209:** 1861, 1969.

2 HERSH, E. M., *et al.:* Hepatotoxic effects of methotrexate. *Cancer,* **19:** 600, 1966.

3 RAGAB, A. H., *et al.:* Osteoporotic fractures secondary to methotrexate therapy of acute leukemia in remission. *Cancer,* **25:** 580, 1970.

4 KAY, H. E. M., *et al.:* Encephalopathy in acute leukemia associated with methotrexate therapy. Arch Dis Child, **47:** 344, 1972.

URIC ACID METABOLISM IN MALIGNANCY

E. FRED SAUNDERS, M.D., F.R.C.P.(C)*

Complications due to uric acid used to be very common in malignancy. In one series of patients with leukemia, 25% had uric acid levels above 12 mg.% at some time during their disease[1]. *Almost* all complications related to uric acid excretion can be prevented. Although hyperuricemia may occur with any malignancy, the difficulties in children arise primarily in association with acute leukemia and lymphosarcoma.

Uric acid is the end product of purine metabolism in man (Table I). In malignancy, cell lysis due to spontaneous cell death or therapy greatly increases

TABLE I

Purine Metabolism

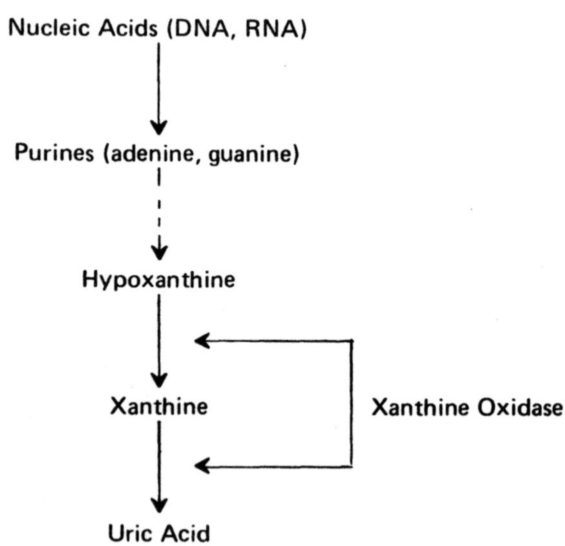

*Staff Hematoligist, The Hospital for Sick Children, Toronto; and Assistant Professor of Pediatrics, University of Toronto.

the production of nucleic acids, and therefore, a great increase in the load of uric acid to be removed from the body. Three-quarters of this uric acid must be secreted by the kidney, yet uric acid is relatively insoluble and crystals tend to precipitate in the distal tubules and collecting system, leading to acute urinary tract obstruction. All attempts at therapy are directed at increasing the solubility of the end products of purine metabolism. In this respect, the final steps in the uric acid formation are most important, because it is here that allopurinol acts. Allopurinol, an analogue of hypoxanthine, has a great affinity for the enzyme, xanthine oxidase. Allopurinol blocks this enzyme and thus reduces the production of uric acid. This action is not complete and purines are excreted as a mixture of hypoxanthine, xanthine and uric acid. Xanthine and hypoxanthine are much more soluble than uric acid. The drug is relatively non-toxic and an occasional allergic rash is the only major side effect.

A number of factors affect deposition of urates in the kidney (Table II) and therapy is based on manipulation of these factors. As already mentioned, allopurinol is used to reduce uric acid levels. Fluids are given to increase urine output. Alkalinization of the urine is important; by increasing urine pH from five to seven, uric-acid solubility is increased 15 times. It is my impression that infiltration of the kidneys by malignancy greatly predisposes to uric-acid nephropathy, and also that patients from families with gout, symptomatic or asymptomatic, have more trouble with uric acid. However, the literature contains no studies on these two points.

TABLE II

Factors in Deposition of Uric Acid Crystals

1. Uric acid levels
2. Urine volume
3. Urine pH
4. Renal infiltration by malignant disease
5. Familial tendency to gout

Complications due to uric acid may present in a number of ways (Table III) of which acute renal shutdown is usually the easiest to recognize. However, the child who presents with vomiting due to oliguria and a slowly rising blood urea nitrogen (BUN), must be distinguished from the patient with central nervous system (CNS) inflitration. If a BUN and uric acid are not done, the diagnosis may be missed, particularly in the outpatient department. Renal colic and acute gout are uncommon. Sinks and his colleagues[2] have reported a syndrome of anorexia, vomiting, drowsiness, lethargy, weakness and convulsions due to hyperuricemia, which must also be distinguished from CNS infiltration.

TABLE III

Presentation of Hyperuricemia

1.	Acute renal shutdown (uric acid nephropathy)
2.	Renal colic (uric acid stones)
3.	Vomiting, drowsiness, lethargy
4.	Acute gout

In most patients therapy is simple. From a review of the leukemias at the Hospital for Sick Children, it was impossible to predict which patients would develop hyperuricemia. There was no direct correlation with blast count, mass of tumor tissue, or the levels of BUN and uric acid on admission. However, patients with very high peripheral blast counts had the greatest risk of uric-acid nephropathy. Therefore, the following regimen was established (Table IV). All patients are routinely treated with prophylactic allopurinol, preferably starting before chemotherapy. For selected cases with white counts over 100,000 or huge masses of lymphosarcoma, bicarbonate and acetazolamide are given to alkalinize the urine. This is advisable because the child still has a uric acid load to excrete and also zanthine stones have been reported recently[3]. The doses quoted are all quite large. Usually five to seven days of allopurinol is sufficient. Alkalinization of the urine can be stopped as soon as the white count falls.

Frequently, it is difficult to administer oral allopurinol to a vomiting child. An intravenous form is available for experimental use, but the dose is unknown. Rectal allopurinol may be used. The dose of tablets is crushed and mixed with 30 cc. of 1% methyl cellulose and instilled into the rectum. A double dose has been recommended but the regular oral dose has been used with success. This is not an approved therapy and no studies have been done of allopurinol blood levels following rectal administration. Nevertheless, this treatment brings uric acid levels down and the patients stay out of trouble.

Because 6-mercaptopurine is degraded by xanthine oxidase, some workers have recommended that the dose of 6-MP be reduced to 1/3 or 1/4 in the presence of allopurinol. However, this is not necessary if allopurinol is given only for a few days.

This program of prophylactic therapy has been so effective that only one child has had renal shutdown in the past two years at the Hospital for Sick Children. Renal shutdown is reversible if treated early and vigorously (Table V). The usual therapy *plus* a trial of mannitol should be given. The fluid load, pH and electrolytes must be carefully monitored. If necessary, peritoneal or hemodialysis can be used. Dialysis is ethical if done early in the disease and there is a reasonable expectation of remission.

TABLE IV

Prophylactic Therapy

Routine	Extraordinary
1. Treat all patients	1. Selected patients
2. Allopurinol 400 $mg/m^2/day$	2. Allopurinol
3. Push fluids	3. $NaHCO_3$ 100 m $equiv/m^2/day$
	4. Acetazolamide 1 $gram/m^2/day$
	5. Push fluids

TABLE V

Therapy of Uric Acid Nephropathy

1. Allopurinol
2. $NaHCO_3$
3. Acetozolamide
4. Mannitol and fluids
5. Peritoneal or hemodialysis

SUMMARY

An increased breakdown of nucleic acids from malignant tissue may produce hyperuricemia. Hyperuricemia can result in renal failure, CNS dysfunction, renal colic or acute gout. These complications can be prevented in almost every case by the routine prophylactic use of allopurinol in children with leukemia and lymphosarcoma. In addition, induction of a diuresis and alkalinization of the urine are occasionally helpful. Allopurinol can be given rectally to the patient who is vomiting.

REFERENCES

1 KRAKOFF, I. H. and MEYER, R. L.: Prevention of hyperuricemia in leukemia and lymphoma. *JAMA*, **193**: 1, 1965.

2 SINKS, L. F., NEWTON, A. W., Jr., NAGI, N. A. and STEVENSON, T. D.: A syndrome associated with extreme hyperuricemia in leukemia. *J Pediatr*, **68**: 578, 1966.

3 BAND, P. R., SILVERBERG, D. S., HENDERSON, J. F., ULAN, R. A., WENSEL, R. H., BANERJEE, T. K. and LITTLE, A. S.: Xanthine nephropathy in a patient with lymphosarcoma treated with allopurinol. *N Engl J Med*. **283**: 354, 1970.

PANEL ON SELECTED PROBLEMS IN MANAGEMENT OF ACUTE LEUKEMIA

Moderator: P. D. McCLURE*
Panelists: P. C. FLEMING**, M. H. FREEDMAN†,
P. J. MIDDLETON‡, E. F. SAUNDERS‡ and
L. F. SINKS††

Dr. D'Angio: I am sure there is such an entity as methotrexate lung but it is always difficult to exclude specific infections and, in particular, *pneumocystis carinii.* How do you rule out infections?

It is curious that continuing therapy with methotrexate will still result in clearing of the lung lesion, unlike bone lesions, for example.

Dr. Freedman: Methotrexate lung is, I feel, still an unproved diagnostic entity. It is always difficult to be sure that the various forms of infectious disease have been excluded. Among the complications of methotrexate therapy, methotrexate lung is the least likely to be due, specifically, to the toxic effect of the drug. Bone toxicity, I think, is well established but lung disease and encephalopathy due to methotrexate are still questionable.

Dr. Sinks: I agree with Dr. Freedman that the nature of methotrexate lung is still obscure. In one of the first ALGB studies with twice-weekly, high-dose methotrexate, there was approximately a 40% incidence of pulmonary complications. Many of these children had lung biopsies. some of which showed fibrosis and an infectious agent could not be isolated, but I agree that the lesion may not represent a direct toxic effect on the alveolar cells. It may be that methotrexate predisposes these tissues to infection with viral or other agents. With regard to bone toxicity, we have investigated three such children by means of intestinal biopsy, bone biopsy and calcium balance studies to locate the defect. On discontinuing methotrexate, all spontaneously improved and suffered no further fractures. Two children developed intracranial calcification, not unlike that seen in the Sturge-Weber syndrome.

---

*The Hospital for Sick Children, Toronto.
**The Hospital for Sick Children, Toronto.
†The Hospital for Sick Children, Toronto.
‡The Hospital for Sick Children, Toronto.
‡The Hospital for Sick Children, Toronto.
††Roswell Park Memorial Institute. Buffalo, N.Y., U.S.A.

Dr. Saunders: A comment on methotrexate lung. It has been suggested that this is a hypersensitivity reaction and that steroids will produce rapid improvement in the radiograph. May I direct a question to Dr. Fleming? He mentioned that pneumocystis infection is commonly seen during periods of remission. I wonder whether recovery from this infection is usually spontaneous? Presently, treatment with pentamidine during relapse or periods of severe immune depression is usually disappointing. "Methotrexate lung" might sometimes be pneumocystis infection which clears spontaneously.

Dr. Fleming: You may be right. Methotrexate acts in the same way as pentamidine – that is, as an inhibitor of the reductase of folic acid. It is possible that you depress the pneumocystis infection during the intensive stage of treatment and that this is released gradually as treatment is discontinued. Pneumocystis infection is related to an impairment in the cellular immune response.

Question: With regard to the prevention of meningeal leukemia, what are the relative merits of intrathecal methotrexate and irradiation?

Dr. Sinks: It does not look as though the results obtained with intrathecal methotrexate will approach those with cerebrospinal irradiation, at least insofar as Dr. Pinkel's results at Memphis are concerned.

Dr. McClure: I wonder whether anyone has any experience with chemical meningitis following intrathecal methotrexate?

Dr. D'Angio: We have had that problem with patients who received methotrexate intraventricularly by way of a shunt. These patients developed what appeared to be mass lesions which, on biopsy, looked like radiation cerebritis, although these patients had received no irradiation. Both of them went on to die. Dr. Caldwell at the Boston Children's Hospital has had a similar experience with intraventricular methotrexate. When it is put in from below, one must guard against what we call the "double-sac syndrome". Patients who have had repeated lumbar punctures develop subdural collections of CSF, which may be quite sizeable and methotrexate may, therefore, be instilled into this sac rather than into the subarachnoid space. This was a possible mechanism in at least one patient who developed the cauda equina syndrome.

Dr. Sinks: Our experience, for some reason, has not been terribly bad. We have all had our share of meningismus induced by intrathecal methotrexate. We have had no severe side effects from intrathecal methotrexate. We have had more arachnoiditis with intrathecal cytosine arabinoside than with intrathecal methotrexate.

Dr. Cowan: In regard to toxicity, may we talk about prednisone and aseptic necrosis of the hip. Drs. Rideout and Alison have collected eight such cases from this institution. All had received steroids, although the interval between steroids and necrosis was as long as 12 months in some patients. One of these patients had acute leukemia. Has Dr. Sinks seen this? In addition, I would like to ask the panel how they feel established meningeal leukemia should be managed in terms of the initial treatment, follow-up and duration of follow-up treatment?

Dr. Sinks: I have nothing to add to the first part of your question. The treatment of established CNS disease is an area of some controversy. The alternatives are intrathecal methotrexate or intrathecal cytosine arabinoside, although now the Southwest group is exploring triple therapy with hydrocortisone, methotrexate and cytosine arabinoside. Then there is craniospinal irradiation. In our hands, high doses of irradiation (about 2400 rads), has not been better than moderate doses in the range of 1000 to 1200 rads. This has also been borne out by Dr. Pinkel's experience at St. Jude's. Curiously enough, we have become almost afraid of these high doses of radiotherapy for established disease, because patients have gone into precipitous bone marrow relapse just after completion of their craniospinal irradiation. At the present time, the most reasonable approach is to use intrathecal methotrexate and a reasonable dose of irradiation, say 1000 to 1200 rads. I am not an advocate of high-dose irradiation for established disease. In contrast, there seems to be little problem associated with 2400 rads when given electively to prevent meningeal leukemia.

Dr. Cowan: What about the frequency and duration of maintenance treatment of meningeal leukemia?

Dr. Sinks: This is very poorly worked out. In a number of patients we have tried giving intrathecal methotrexate on a monthly basis following control of meningeal leukemia, but this has not prevented relapse. We do not have a controlled study on this, however. To my knowledge, at present, there is no good way of maintaining a patient in CNS remission.

Dr. Saunders: My feelings are rather different. One thing that children really hate is a needle and we try to approach this so they get as few needles as possible. In established CNS disease, it has been our practice to treat CNS symptoms only. Usually, we start with intrathecal methotrexate and if we can get away with one good-sized injection, we do so. We do not repeat it until the child has further symptoms. Sometimes one dose may be adequate for three to six months. If they are given monthly injections, they end up with a tremendous number of lumbar punctures with no guarantee of preventing a relapse of their CNS disease.

Question: You have indicated that a high percentage of leukemic patients develop episodes of fever with suspected septicemia. If this is not proven by positive blood cultures or other adequately taken cultures, how long do you think therapy should be continued?

Dr. Fleming: If it is not proven by, say three days, by blood culture, there are a number of possibilities. First, that there is an organism, which takes longer to grow or an organism, which is not even being cultured for, such as mycoplasma, or, as a rare possibility, you may be dealing with a fungal infection, which will not come up until later. After three days you should certainly consider adding amphotericin to the drug regimen. When to stop, is difficult. In many clinical situations, after five days of polyvalent antibacterial therapy without response, it would be reasonable to stop all these drugs and reinvestigate the patient with blood and other cultures.

Dr. Sinks: May I comment on that? This is a very controversial area. First of all, and I am sure you meant to imply this, one has to address oneself to the stage of the disease. The pattern of infections when the child is initially admitted is very different from that in the late-stage, suppressed patient with granulocytopenia. In a recent review of our material by Dr. Arnold Freedman, we found that about one-third of the patients over the last several years had autopsy evidence of Candida infection. Most of these children had mixed infections. Escherichia coli was slightly commoner than pseudomonas.

It is extremely difficult to rescue the terminal patient, who is always leukopenic and granulocytopenic, without anticipating either white-cell transfusions or an impending remission with chemotherapy. Because, if you do not get some leukocytes in by one method or another, you can give all the antibiotics you want and you will probably not retrieve them. We have been relying to some extent on white-cell transfusions but this is still not satisfactory. You have to give them substantial amounts on repeated occasions, otherwise they are worthless. I would like to comment as well on gut sterilization in children and the "life island". The only control study in the United States of the life island and its effect is being conducted at Roswell Park. These are adult patients with myeloblastic leukemia who have been randomized with and without gut sterilization in the life island. The results at this time are not very encouraging because we see no benefit from the more extensive procedure. In children, there is no place for gut sterilization at this particular time. They go into remission rapidly and do not succumb to the gram-negative organisms.

Dr. Fleming: I am very pleased to hear that, and I quite agree with you about the life island. I do not think it has a place in pediatric work. I did not wish to imply that you discontinue antifungal agents after a two-day trial. I was referring to the antibacterial agents alone.

Dr. Saunders: What percentage of blood cultures are positive in this group of patients?

Dr. Fleming: A relatively small proportion approximately 20%. In a recent review, we did not have a single positive culture in a patient who had more than 1000 granulocytes. All the positive cultures were in the children with severe granulocytopenia, even though all the patients tended to look the same; they had fever and appeared to be septic. The antileukemic chemotherapy may depress the retrieval rate of blood cultures. Whilst we have not noted any correlation between the antileukemic therapy, the granulocyte count, and the frequency of positive blood cultures, we have not investigated this in a prospective fashion.

INDEX

actinomycin-D
adverse effects of, 40
influence on metastases, 34-39
influence on recurrence rate, 37-39
influence on survival rate, 35-39
in treatment of ovarian tumors, 79
in treatment of rhabdomyosarcoma, 165-194
in treatment of Wilms' tumor, 17, 18, 34-40, 49, 55-59
Acute Leukemia Group B, 216-224
adenocarcinoma of testis 60-77. *See also* metastases
chemotherapy for, 70, 72, 74, 75
description of, 61, 68
lymphadenectomy for, 69-76
mortality rate for. 72, 73
occurrence of, 70
orchidectomy for, 61, 68, 70, 72-75
radiotherapy for, 61, 70, 72, 74, 75
survival rate for, 61, 63, 70, 72
Adriamycin (doxorubicin)
in treatment of non-Hodgkin's lymphoma, 206
in treatment of rhabdomyosarcoma, 194
androgen therapy. *See* nasopharyngeal angiofibroma
anemia
with neuroblastoma. 171
antigens, tumor-specific
and neuroblastoma, 180-183, 195-196
antitumor immunity, 180-183. *See also* Hellstrom
bacterial infections, 229-232. *See also* leukemia, acute

BCNU
in treatment of medulloblastoma, 110-111
Beckwith, J. Bruce, 49-54
Bishop, Harry C., 49-54
bleomycin
in treatment of neuroblastoma, 175
brain, tumors of, 83-84, 108-112. *See also* cerebrospinal fluid cytology. diabetes insipidus; neuroradiology
chemotherapy for. 110-111
radiotherapy for. 108, 110-111
sites of, 84
symptoms of, 83, 85, 86
types of, 83-84
Breslow, Norman. 49-54
Burkitt. D. P., 209-213, 214-215
Burkitt's lymphoma. 205, 209-213. *See also* immunology
age distribution of, 209-210
chemotherapy for, 212, 213
and EB virus, 211, 212, 215
geographical distribution of, 209-212
identification of. 209-210, 215
and malaria. 211-212
survival rate for, 212

Canadian Tumor Reference Centre, 60, 64
cancer
age-specific death rate for, 6-9
age-specific incidence rate for, 10
as cause of death, 5, 6
lethal sites of, 6-7
sex difference incidence of, 6, 10-12, 21, 23
carcinoma myxomatodes. *See* adenocarcinoma of testis
cerebrospinal fluid cytology
in diagnosis of brain tumors, 108-109
chemotherapy. *See* adenocarcinoma of testis; brain, tumors of; Burkitt's lymphoma; hyperuricemia; hystiocytosis X; leukemia; malignant liver tumor; malignant ovarian tumor; medulloblastoma; nasopharyngeal angiofibroma; neuroblastoma; non-Hodgkin's lymphoma; rhabdomyosarcoma; Wilm's tumor.
chlorambucil
in treatment of neuroblastoma. 17
corpus callosum, 87-88, 91
effects of incision of, 109
cortisone
in treatment of Wilms' tumor. 17, 18
cyclophosphamide
in treatment of histiocytosis X, 133
in treatment of neuroblastoma, 17, 175
in treatment of non-Hodgkin's lymphoma, 206
in treatment of rhabdomyosarcoma. 165, 194
in treatment of stage IV^S neuroblastoma, 175
in treatment of Wilms' tumor, 17, 18
cytosine arabinoside
in treatment of leukemia. 241-242
cytoxan
in treatment of neuroblastoma, 192

Dandy's approach. *See* posterior third ventricle tumors
D'Angio, Guilio J., 49-54, 55-59, 185, 191-198, 214, 240-241
Darte J. M. M., 30, 55-59, 191-198, 199-201
daunomycin
in treatment of neuroblastoma, 175
daunorubicin
in treatment of leukemia. 217-219
Decadron (dexamethasone)
in treatment of medulloblastoma, 110
Deltacortisone. *See* prednisone
Dent, Peter B., 179-184, 191-198, 214
diabetes insipidus
with histiocytosis X, 120, 122, 131, 134
with posterior third ventricle tumors. 103-105
as symptoms of brain tumor, 85, 86
doxorubicon. *See* Adriamycin

INDEX

EB virus. *See* Burkitt's lymphoma
and infectious mononucleosis, 211
Ein, Sigmund H., 78-82, 166-170
embryonal adenocarcinoma. *See* adenocarcinoma of testis
embryonal carcinoma. *See* adenocarcinoma of testis
endodermal sinus tumor. *See* adenocarcinoma of testis
eosinophilic granuloma. *See* histiocytosis X
Evans, Audrey E., 49-54, 185, 192
fetal mesodermal hamartoma. *See* hamartoma, fetal mesodermal

Fitzpatrick, P. J., 139-156
Fleming, P. C., 229-232, 240-244
Freedman, M. H., 233-235, 240-244
fungal infections. *See* leukemia, acute

Ghavimi, F., 128-138
Goodwin, Willard E., 49-54
hamartoma, fetal mesodermal, 42-48. *See also* metastases; pathology
description of, 42-45
survival rate for, 47
symptoms of, 42
treatment of, 45, 47-48

Hand-Schüller-Christian syndrome, 125
Harwood-Nash, Derek, 92-97, 108-112
Hellstrom, K. E. and I.
and antitumor immunity, 179-182
Hendrick, E. Bruce, 83-84, 85-91, 108-112
histiocytic lymphoma. *See* non-Hodgkin's lymphoma
histiocytosis X, 113-127, 128-138. *See also* diabetes insipidus; Hand-Schüller-Christian syndrome; Letterer-Siwe syndrome
and eosinophilic granuloma, 113, 117-120, 125, 126
extraskeletal lesions in, 120, 126
incidence of, 113-127
and lesions of liver, 122-123
and lesions of lung, 125
and lesions of lymph nodes, 122, 126
and lesions of pituitary, 120-122
and lesions of skin, 122, 124
and lesions of spleen, 122, 124
and lesions of thymus, 125
pathology of, 113-127
sites of, 115-116
skeletal lesions in, 117, 126
histiocytosis X, multiple system, 128, 131-137
chemotherapy for, 132-133
radiotherapy for, 128, 132, 134
surgery for, 128
survival rate for, 135-138
symptoms of, 131
histiocytosis X, single system, 128-131
radiotherapy for, 128-131
recurrence rate for, 129-131
surgery for, 128-130
survival rate for, 131
Hodgkin's disease, 202-203
diagnosis of extent of, 202
laparotomy in staging of, 202-203
mortality rate for, 7-9
radiology in diagnosis of, 202
Hoffman, H. J., 85-91, 108-112
Horner's syndrome, 172
hyperuricemia, 236-239. *See also* leukemia, acute
causes of, 237
complications due to, 236-237
treatment of, 237, 238

immunodepression
and viral infections, 227-228
immunology, 179-184. *See also* Hellstrom
and Burkitt's lyphoma, 211-213
and neuroblastoma, 171, 176, 179-183
immunosuppression
and actinomycin-D, 40
and methotrexate, 234-235
and viral infections, 225-227
infectious mononucleosis, 211

Jeffs, Robert D., 55-59, 68-77
Jenkins, R.D.T., 55-59, 108-112, 157-165

Kikuchi, J., 199-201
King, Lowell R., 48-54
Koop, C. Everett, 185-190, 191-198

laparotomy
in Hodgkin's disease, 202-203, 214
of neuroblastoma, 176, 191
of non-Hodgkin's lymphoma, 205, 215
of ovarian tumors, 79, 81
L-asparaginase
in treatment of leukemia. 217-219
leiomyoma of the kidney. *See* hamartoma, fetal mesodermal
Letterer-Siwe syndrome. 113, 125
leukemia, 216-232
controlled clinical trials in, 216-224
incidence of, 10
mortality rate for, 7
psychological effects of, 199
types of, 23
leukemia, acute, 216-232. *See also* Leukemia Group B
bacterial infections with, 229-232
chemotherapy for. 216-219, 241-242
and complications due to uric acid, 236-238
fungal infections with, 229
and hyperuricemia, 236-238
and methotrexate lung, 234-236
survival rate for. 219-224
viral infections with, 225-228

leukemia, meningeal, 241-242
effects of methotrexate on, 241-241
radiotherapy for, 242
leukemic transformation
in non-Hodgkin's lymphoma, 205
liver tumors. *See* malignant liver tumors
lymphadenectomy *See* adenocarcinoma of testis
lymphoma of testis. *See* malignant lymphoma of testis
lymphosarcoma. *See* Manchester Children's Tumor Registry; non-Hodgkin's lymphoma; uric acid

MacKay, E. N., 5-20
Magner, Desmond, 60-67, 68
malignant liver tumors, 166-170. *See also* metastases, lung
chemotherapy for, 168
diagnosis of, 166-167, 169
pathology of, 167
radiotherapy for, 168
surgery for, 168-169
survival rate for, 166
symptoms of, 166
types of, 167
malignant lymphoma of testis, 64-66
malignant ovarian tumors, 78-82. *See also* metastases
chemotherapy for, 79-82
diagnosis of, 81-82
pathology of, 78-74
radiotherapy for, 79-82
surgery for, 79, 81-82
survival rate for, 80
symptoms of, 78
types of, 78-79
Mancer, J. F. K., 42-48, 113-127
Manchester Children's Tumor Registry, 21-28
lymphosarcoma recorded at, 24
nephroblastoma recorded at, 24, 28
neuroblastoma recorded at, 24
and renal tumors, 24-25
retinoblastomas recorded at, 24-25
treatments used, 18, 28
types of leukemia recorded at, 23
McClure, P. D., 214-215, 240-244
McLerie, E. E., 5-20
medulloblastoma. *See also* metastases
chemotherapy for, 110-111
extent of, 15
incidence of, 12, 13
radiotherapy for, 17, 111-112
surgery for, 17, 111-112
survival rate for, 13-17, 20
6-mercaptopurine
in treatment of hyperuricemia, 238
in treatment of leukemia. 218-219
metastases
with adenocarcinoma of testis, 72, 74, 75
with fetal mesodermal hamartoma, 47
with malignant ovarian tumors, 78-81
with medulloblastoma, 15
with neonatal Wilms' tumor, 46
with neuroblastoma, 12, 15, 171-176, 186-187
with rhabdomyosarcoma, 159, 165
with testicular tumors, 61, 63, 65
with Wilms' tumor, 15, 31, 35-40, 50, 55, 59
metastases, of bone and bone marrow
with neuroblastoma, 171-176, 186-187, 192-193
with stage IV^S neuroblastoma, 192-193
metastases, lung, 18, 31, 32, 34-36, 38-40
with malignant liver tumors, 167-169
with medulloblastoma, 17, 18
with neuroblastoma, 17, 18, 171
with Wilms' tumor. 50, 55
methotrexate
with brain tumors, 110
with histiocytosis X, 122, 133, 135
with leukemia, 216-220, 240-243
with medulloblastoma, 110
toxic effects of, 233-235, 241
methotrexate lung, 234, 240-241
with leukemia, 234-236
with liver disease, 234
methotrexate toxicity, 233-235
with histiocytosis X, 122, 135
symptoms of, 233-234
Middleton, Peter J., 225-228, 240-244
Morris-Jones, P. H., 21-28
Mott, Martin, 204-208

nasopharyngeal angiofibroma, 139-156
androgen therapy for, 145, 154
diagnostic radiology for, 142-145, 153
pathology for, 139-140
radiotherapy for, 139, 145-156
recurrence rate for, 145
surgery for, 145, 147
National Wilms' Tumor Study Group, 31, 49-54
neonatal renal tumors, 42-48. *See also* hamartoma, fetal mesodermal; Wilms' tumor
nephroblastoma. *See* Manchester Children's Tumor Registry
nephroma, congenital mesoblastic. *See* hamartoma, fetal mesodermal
neuroblastoma, 171-178. *See also* anemia; immunology; Horner's syndrome; Manchester Children's Tumor Registry; metastases; Pepper's syndrome
biochemical investigation of, 172-173
chemotherapy for, 17, 174-175, 186-187, 189, 194-195
diagnosis of, 171-172
incidence of, 12
radiotherapy for, 17, 174-176, 185-189, 195, 197-198
sites of, 15, 171-172, 196
staging system for, 185-187, 190
surgery for, 17, 174-175, 185-189, 197
survival rate for, 12-15, 17, 19, 24, 25
symptoms of, 173, 174
neuroblastoma, stage IV^S, 175-176, 187, 189, 191-195, 198

chemotherapy for, 191, 192
radiotherapy for, 191, 192
surgery for, 192-195
neuroradiology
by angiogram, 92-95, 109
of brain tumors, 109
by pneumoencephalogram, 94-97
of posterior third ventricle tumors, 92-97, 103
by ventriculogram, 92-94, 109
nitrogen mustard
in treatment of neuroblastoma, 17, 192
in treatment of Wilms' tumor, 17
non-Burkitt's lymphoma, 205-207
non-Burkitt's lymphoma (lymphosarcoma), 204-208
chemotherapy for, 206-207
classification of, 204-205
difficulty in diagnosis of, 204-205
radiotherapy for, 206-207
sites of, 205
survival rate for, 206
Norman, M. G., 98-101, 108-112

Ontario Cancer Incidence Survey, 10
operative treatment
for neuroblastoma, 185-189
for rhabdomyosarcoma, 189-190
orchidectomy. *See* adenocarcinoma of testis; testicular tumors
orchioblastoma. *See* adenocarcinoma of testis.
ovarian tumors. *See* malignant ovarian tumors

Pakes, E. H., 199-201
paratesticular sarcoma, 60-63, 65-66
pathology. *See also* malignant liver tumors; malignant ovarian tumors
of fetal mesodermal hamartoma, 42
of histiocytosis X, 113-127
of posterior third ventricle masses, 98-101
of tumors of testis, 60-67
Pepper's syndrome, 172, 175
Pickett, Lawrence K., 49-54
pineal tumors. *See* teratomas in pineal region
posterior third ventricle tumors, 85-107
abnormalities in, 96
case histories of, 86-89
characteristics of, 94
Dandy's approach, 85-86, 91
mortality rate for, 85, 89
neuroradiological investigation of, 92-97, 103
pathology of, 98-101
radiotherapy for. 85-87, 91, 102-107
sites of, 93
surgery for, 102, 106-107, 111
surgical approaches for, 85-86
survival rate for, 86, 104, 105
Torkildsen shunt, 85-86, 91
ventriculoperitoneal shunt, 85-87, 89
prednisone (deltacortisone)
in treatment of aseptic necrosis of hip, 241-242
in treatment of histiocytosis X, 133
in treatment of leukemia, 216-219
in treatment of, non-Hodgkin's lymphoma, 206
procarbazine
in treatment of neuroblastoma, 175
psychiatric problems, 199-200

radiology, 142-145. *See also* Hodgkin's disease; nasopharyngeal angiofibroma
radiotherapy. *See also* adenocarcinoma of testis; brain tumors; histiocytosis X; leukemia; malignant liver tumors; malignant ovarian tumors; medulloblastoma; neuroblastoma; non-Hodgkin's lymphoma; rhabdomyosarcoma; Wilms' tumor
and methotrexate, 241-242
of nasopharyngeal angiofibroma, 139-156
of posterior third ventricle tumors, 102-107
renal tumors. *See* hamartoma, fetal mesodermal; Manchester Children's Tumor Registry
rhabdomyosarcoma, 157-165. *See also* metastases
chemotherapy for, 165, 189-190, 194-195
and interstitial implantation, 196-197
occurrence of, 157
radiotherapy for, 161-165, 189-190
recurrence rate for, 159
site of, 157, 158
staging scheme for, 189
surgery for, 161, 165, 189-190, 195
survival rate for, 157, 159, 160
of testis, 60, 63, 66
Rider, W. D., 139-156

Saunders, E. Fred, 214, 236-239, 240-244
Schweisguth, Odile, 58-59, 111-112, 171-178, 191-198, 215
Sellers, A. H., 5-20
Sinks, Lucius F., 49-54, 196, 216-224, 237, 240-244
Sonley, M. J., 29-41, 55-59, 108-112, 128-138, 198, 199-201
Stephens, Clinton A., 166-170, 191-198, 202-203, 214-215
Sullivan, Margaret, 204-208
surgery. *See* adenocarcinoma of testis; histiocytosis X; Hodgkin's disease; malignant liver tumors, malignant ovarian tumors; medulloblastoma; nasopharyngeal angiofibroma; neuroblastoma; non-Hodgkin's lymphoma; posterior third ventricle tumors; rhabdomyosarcoma; testicular tumors; Wilms' tumor
Sutow, Wataru W., 49-54, 204-208

teratomas
  malignant ovarian, 79-81
  in pineal region, 85-89, 98, 103-106
  of testis, 64
testicular tumors, 60-77. *See also* adenocarcinoma of testis; metastases
  description of, 61
  incidence of, 60, 68
  orchidectomy for, 61, 63-66
  pathology of, 60-67
Torkildsen shunt. *See* posterior third ventricle tumor

uric acid. *See also* hyperuricemia; leukemia, acute
  metabolism of in malignancy, 236-239

ventriculoperitoneal shunt. *See* posterior third ventricle tumor
vinblastine sulfate
  in treatment of histiocytosis X, 133
vincoleukoblastine
  in treatment of histiocytosis X, 133
vincristine
  in treatment of histiocytosis X, 133
  in treatment of leukemia, 216-219
  in treatment of medulloblastoma, 110-111
  in treatment of neuroblastoma, 17, 175, 192
  in treatment of non-Hodgkin's lymphoma, 206
  in treatment of rhabdomyosarcoma, 165, 194
  in treatment of stage IV^S neuroblastoma, 175
  in treatment of Wilms' tumor, 40, 49, 55-59
viral infections, 225-228. *See also* leukemia, acute
  risk of from immunodepression, 227-228
  risk of from immunosuppression, 225-227
  treatment of, 226-227

Wilbur, Jordan R., 58-59, 110, 191-198, 204-208, 214-215
Wilms' tumor, 29-41, 49-59. *See also* metastases
  chemotherapy for, 17, 18, 32-41, 49, 50, 55-59
  classification of, 31, 50-52
  incidence of, 12
  neonatal, 42, 46
  radiotherapy for, 17, 30, 32-35, 40-41, 49-52, 56-59
  recurrence rate for, 37-40, 56-57
  sites of, 15
  surgery for, 17, 32-33, 41, 49, 58-59
  survival rate for, 13-17, 20, 32-40, 58
Wolff, James A., 49-54

yolk sac tumor. *See* adenocarcinoma of testis

GPSR Compliance

The European Union's (EU) General Product Safety Regulation (GPSR) is a set of rules that requires consumer products to be safe and our obligations to ensure this.

If you have any concerns about our products, you can contact us on ProductSafety@springernature.com

In case Publisher is established outside the EU, the EU authorized representative is:

Springer Nature Customer Service Center GmbH
Europaplatz 3
69115 Heidelberg, Germany

Batch number: 10620163

Printed by Printforce, the Netherlands